Practical Issues in Geriatrics

Series Editor
Stefania Maggi
Aging Branch
CNR-Neuroscience Institute
Padua, Italy

This practically oriented series presents state of the art knowledge on the principal diseases encountered in older persons and addresses all aspects of management, including current multidisciplinary diagnostic and therapeutic approaches. It is intended as an educational tool that will enhance the everyday clinical practice of both young geriatricians and residents and also assist other specialists who deal with aged patients. Each volume is designed to provide comprehensive information on the topic that it covers, and whenever appropriate the text is complemented by additional material of high educational and practical value, including informative video-clips, standardized diagnostic flow charts and descriptive clinical cases. Practical Issues in Geriatrics will be of value to the scientific and professional community worldwide, improving understanding of the many clinical and social issues in Geriatrics and assisting in the delivery of optimal clinical care.

Lee Smith · Igor Grabovac
Editors

Sexual Behaviour and Health in Older Adults

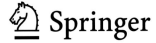

Editors
Lee Smith
Center for Health Performance and
Wellbeing
Anglia Ruskin University
Cambridge, UK

Igor Grabovac
Department of Social and Preventive
Medicine
Centre for Public Health, Medical
University of Vienna
Vienna, Austria

ISSN 2509-6060 ISSN 2509-6079 (electronic)
Practical Issues in Geriatrics
ISBN 978-3-031-21028-0 ISBN 978-3-031-21029-7 (eBook)
https://doi.org/10.1007/978-3-031-21029-7

© Springer Nature Switzerland AG 2023
This work is subject to copyright. All rights are reserved by the Publisher, whether the whole or part of the material is concerned, specifically the rights of translation, reprinting, reuse of illustrations, recitation, broadcasting, reproduction on microfilms or in any other physical way, and transmission or information storage and retrieval, electronic adaptation, computer software, or by similar or dissimilar methodology now known or hereafter developed.
The use of general descriptive names, registered names, trademarks, service marks, etc. in this publication does not imply, even in the absence of a specific statement, that such names are exempt from the relevant protective laws and regulations and therefore free for general use.
The publisher, the authors, and the editors are safe to assume that the advice and information in this book are believed to be true and accurate at the date of publication. Neither the publisher nor the authors or the editors give a warranty, expressed or implied, with respect to the material contained herein or for any errors or omissions that may have been made. The publisher remains neutral with regard to jurisdictional claims in published maps and institutional affiliations.

This Springer imprint is published by the registered company Springer Nature Switzerland AG
The registered company address is: Gewerbestrasse 11, 6330 Cham, Switzerland

Preface

Aging is a global phenomenon. It has been well established that the population of persons over 60 years of age is rapidly growing, making this age group the fastest growing population worldwide. However, longer life expectancy does not also mean that people are living healthier lives. This is seen as a rise in prevalence of chronic diseases as well as neurocognitive issues such as dementia. Overall, years spent in good health have stayed relatively constant, meaning that the additional years gained by the rise in life expectancy are spent in poor health. Therefore, the focus of health practitioners as well as policy makers should turn to health promoting and preventive interventions focusing on improving physical, mental, and social health with an emphasis on healthy aging. This also needs to include sexual health and well-being.

It is a common misconception that older adults do not engage in sexual activities. However, epidemiological studies, including analyses of various nationally representative data, show that older adults engage in sexual activities on a regular basis. What does change with aging is the frequency of sexual activities and activities performed, with shared intimacy including kissing, petting, and mutual masturbation being more common than oral, vaginal, or anal intercourse. More common knowledge is that of physical, mental, and social health influencing sexual activity in older adults; however less research is done to show if and how sexual activities influence health. Emerging research in this field indicates that sexual activities have a wide variety of positive effects on the health and well-being of older adults.

This book is primarily aimed at specialists in geriatrics and all those interested in gerontology and working with older adults. Additionally, it would be of interest to all healthcare professionals working with older adults, as well as those doing research in aging and sexual health. The book is comprised of 15 chapters which showcase how vibrant and active the fields of sexual health and geriatrics are confirming that good work in these fields is only possible through multidisciplinary approaches. This book has been achieved by a group of coauthors from a variety of fields including general medicine, geriatrics and gerontology, psychology, public health, nursing, occupational therapy, social science, sport and nutritional science. The chapters cover a variety of issues from epidemiological analyses and aging in general to specifics on how health influences sexual activities and vice versa. Additionally, the book contains chapters focusing on implementation and practical work outlining barriers and facilitators for sexual activity in older adults as well as questions of promotion of these topics in everyday work and practical issues on communication with patients.

What has been a common theme throughout the book is the lack of research in this field, given the misconceptions and assumptions of asexuality in older adults. It is our hope that the first edition of this book provides an overview of the topic and inspires a new generation of practitioners and researchers to do more projects and continue to contribute to this field.

Cambridge, UK Lee Smith
Vienna, Austria Igor Grabovac

Acknowledgments

The authors wish to thank all the coauthors, who selflessly contributed their time and expertise for this book. On a personal note, we also would like to thank our families for their constant support.

Professor Lee Smith & Dr. Igor Grabovac

Contents

1 **Introduction**... 1
  Sandra Haider and Igor Grabovac

2 **Levels and Trends of Sexual Activity in Older Adults**............... 9
  Guillermo F. López-Sánchez, José M. Oliva-Lozano, José
  M. Muyor, and Lee Smith

3 **Sexual Activity and Physical Health Benefits in Older Adults**....... 15
  Pinar Soysal and Esin Avsar

4 **Sexual Activity and Mental Health Benefits in Older Adults**......... 25
  Tobias Schiffler, Hanna M. Mües, and Igor Grabovac

5 **Sexual Activity and Psychosocial Benefits in Older
  Adults: Challenges and Ways Forward**............................... 45
  Siniša Grabovac and Radhika Seiler-Ramadas

6 **'We're Still Here, We're Still Queer, We're Still
  Doing It': Sex and Sexual Health in Older LGBTQ+ Adults**......... 59
  Joshua W. Katz, Lee Smith, and Daragh T. McDermott

7 **Risky Sexual Activity and Its Impact on Mental
  and Physical Health in Older Adults**.............................. 77
  Daragh T. McDermott and Igor Grabovac

8 **Lifelong Sexual Practice and Its Influence on Health
  in Later Life**... 93
  Benny Rana, Lin Yang, and Siniša Grabovac

9 **Medication Use and Sexual Activity in Older Adults**................ 105
  Damiano Pizzol, Petre Cristian Ilie, and Nicola Veronese

10 **Barriers to Sexual Activity in Older Adults**....................... 113
   Nicola Veronese and Damiano Pizzol

11 **Lifestyle Factors Supporting and Maintaining Sexual
   Activity in Older Adults**... 119
   Sandra Haider, Angela Schwarzinger, and Thomas Ernst Dorner

12	**Promotion of Sex in Older Adults** 139	
	Hanna M. Mües, Kathrin Kirchheiner, and Igor Grabovac	
13	**Future Directions for Research and Practice in Sexual Health for Older Adults** 157	
	Igor Grabovac	
14	**Concluding Summary** 169	
	Igor Grabovac and Lee Smith	
15	**Glossary** 175	
	Lisa Lehner and Charlotte Rösel	

Introduction

1

Sandra Haider and Igor Grabovac

1.1 The Ageing Population

With some exceptions, the worldwide population is ageing and people are living longer. Therefore, both the size of the population and the proportion of older persons are growing. When examining data published by the World Health Organization (WHO) [1], by 2030, one in six people in the world will be ≥60 years, and by 2050, the world's population of people ≥60 years will be approximately 22%. Additionally, the number of persons aged ≥80 years is expected to triple by 2050. This shift towards older ages, known as "population ageing", has already started in high-income countries and is now strongly represented in low- and middle-income countries. Due to this demographic shift, countries are having to adapt their public health systems and implement changes to their social care provision in order to meet this growing demand.

1.2 Living Healthy Lives: Successful Ageing

A longer life brings with it opportunities for the people and their families personally, and also for the society. The extent of these opportunities depends heavily on people's health. However, evidence shows that the proportion of life in good health has remained broadly constant, meaning that the additional years alive are predominantly spent in poor health [2]. For example, data from the European Union (EU) collected in 2020 highlighted that the number of healthy life years was estimated at 64.5 years for women and 63.5 years for men, respectively. This represents only

---

S. Haider · I. Grabovac (✉)
Department of Social and Preventive Medicine, Center for Public Health, Medical University of Vienna, Vienna, Austria
e-mail: sandra.a.haider@meduniwien.ac.at; igor.grabovac@meduniwien.ac.at

© Springer Nature Switzerland AG 2023
L. Smith, I. Grabovac (eds.), *Sexual Behaviour and Health in Older Adults*, Practical Issues in Geriatrics, https://doi.org/10.1007/978-3-031-21029-7_1

77.6% and 81.9% of the total life expectancy for women and men [3]. That is why it is no longer just about living longer, but also about maintaining a healthy quality of life. In this context, the term "successful ageing" is important to consider, which includes, according to the classic concept of Rowe and Kahn, high physical, psychological, and social functioning without major diseases [3].

Lifestyle factors are modifiable factors that can be used to promote and maintain an independent life and can as such contribute to the successful ageing. Such factors include among others levels of social support, regular physical activity, a balanced diet, low levels of smoking behaviour, and regulated alcohol intake. All these factors have been shown to improve and sustain good levels of physical and mental activity, delay care dependency, reduce the risk of non-communicable diseases, and prevent the onset of geriatric syndrome of frailty, an issue which we will explore in more detail.

1.3 Change with Ageing

Within the ageing process, a gradual decrease in physiological reserve occurs, including physical but also mental changes. More in-depth analyses of the physiology of ageing may be found in appropriate texts; however, inspired by Taylor and colleagues [4] we provide a summarized list of some of the core changes that occur. These include physiological, cardiovascular, and musculoskeletal changes that when combined can lead to a deterioration of overall physical and psychological functioning. They include:

Physiological changes

- ↓ vital capacity
- ↓ renal function
- ↓ nerve conduction velocity
- ↓ basal metabolism
- ↓ isoimmunity
- mitochondrial dysfunction,
- cellular senescence,
- endocrine and hormonal change.

Muscle changes

- ↓ muscle mass
- ↓ muscle strength
- ↓ number of fast-twitch fibres
- ↓ physical performance and fitness (including the coordinative skills balance, reaction time, etc.)

Changes in the cardiovascular system

- ↓ oxygen uptake
- ↓ maximum heart rate.

Further changes

- ↓ senses (hearing, seeing, tasting, touching, smelling)
- ↑ swallowing and chewing difficulties
- ↑ loneliness and isolation (due to functional limitations and the restricted ability to maintain relationships outside).

Owing to these changes, chronic diseases become more common.

- ↑ hypertension, high cholesterol, arteriosclerosis, ischaemic heart disease, heart failure
- ↑ arthritis, osteoporosis, hip fractures
- ↑ stroke, Parkinson's disease
- ↑ diabetes type 2
- ↑ cancer
- ↑ incontinence
- ↑ dementia, Alzheimer's disease
- ↑ depression
- ↑ chronic kidney disease
- ↑ chronic obstructive pulmonary disease.

1.4 The Geriatric Syndrome Frailty

As described above, a gradual decrease in physiological reserves is a normal process associated with the ageing process. However, when this decline is accelerated and homeostatic mechanisms are restricted, the geriatric syndrome of frailty appears [5]. According to the definition by Fried and colleagues, a definition that is widely acknowledged as being the most comprehensive, frailty is characterized by an increased vulnerability to external stressors and is based on the five predefined physical criteria, namely: (1) weight loss, (2) exhaustion, (3) low physical activity, (4) slowness, and (5) weakness [6].

In an ageing population, frailty is very common. As such, data indicates that the prevalence of frailty and prefrailty among the European community-dwelling population of older adults is estimated to be 50.6% [7]. As frailty is increasingly prevalent and as it is associated with various age-related declines, for example, increased vulnerability, disabilities, a greater likelihood of falls, morbidity, hospitalization, nursing home admission, dependency, and mortality [8–10]. These factors combine to reduce an elderly persons quality of life and with reduced healthy life years, the associated increased dependence results in greater costs to both social care and health systems [5, 11, 12].

Therefore, the efforts to avoid or deter the onset of frailty should be made so as to enable successful ageing. For this purpose, key lifestyle interventions can be recommended as well as regular physical activity, a balanced diet, and social support can help delay the onset of frailty.

1.5 Sexual Activity and Ageing

A common misconception among clinicians and researchers is that older adults do not engage in sexual activities and there is often a mistaken assumption of elderly asexuality. However, epidemiological data suggests that even as there is a marked decline in sexual activity with age, older adults are still sexually active, with the proportions being relatively high even among very old adults. For example a study by Lindau et al. reported that among older adults aged 75–85 who reported some sexual activity, 54% reported engaging in sexual activity 2–3 times a month, with almost 25% reporting weekly sexual activities [13]. For more details on the prevalence of sexual activities in this population, please see Chap. 2. What is important to note are the changes in the importance that older adults place on sexual activity, as studies note that older men place more importance on sexual activity compared to older women.

Overall when considering sexual activity in older adults, we need to consider that sex includes a variety of activities, which may include touching, petting, kissing, masturbation, exchanging of fantasies as well as penetrative (oral, vaginal, or anal) sex. Overall data on sexual activities among older adults are scarce and limited due to a lack of systematic coverage of this topic among clinical and academic researchers. Of the data that is available, these are often limited by factors such as the use of convenience sampling methods and are almost exclusively conducted with cisgender (i.e., people whose self-identified gender identity aligns with their biological sex as assigned at birth) and heterosexual participants [14]. With this in mind, the most common form of sexual activity reported by older adults is vaginal intercourse reported by 80% of men and 75% of women aged 75–85 years [15, 16].

1.6 Health and Sexual Activity in Older Adults

With increased age there is also a rise in prevalence of chronic illnesses and multimorbidities [17], all of which can directly impact the frequency of a persons' sexual activity and an overall satisfying sex life. This is important as sustaining good health is a key component of maintaining sexual activities across the life span. Some studies have demonstrated that older adults who experience good or excellent self-reported health also report greater frequency and higher levels of satisfaction with their levels of sexual activity. Chronic illness on the other hand can reduce mobility, detrimentally influence mood, and lower a persons' desire for sex and also reduce self-esteem often leading to a decline in sexual function and decrease in the frequency of sexual activity. For example, type 2 diabetes mellitus and arterial hypertension both are associated with endothelial dysfunction which may lead to erectile dysfunction in older men, while arthritis is a major cause of disability in both older men and women and may also interfere with sexual activity and function due to pain and joint stiffness [18]. For a more detailed examination of the relationship between physical health and sexual activity, please see Chap. 3.

Aside from the effects of various chronic illnesses that increase in prevalence as a person ages, a range of physiological changes also affect sexual health in both older men and women. Following puberty, for women, the most important period for sexual and reproductive health is menopause, which occurs due to a decrease in the ovarian production of oestradiol and progesterone as well as changes in the release of follicle-stimulating hormone and oestrogen. The experienced drop in the production of these hormones has an effect on all organ systems causing a variety of physiological changes. In terms of sexual well-being, menopause is often associated with dyspareunia (i.e., pain during sexual intercourse) and decrease of vaginal lubrication [19]. While men do experience a drop in the production of testosterone, possibly due to loss of testicular function as well as hypothalamic dysregulation, the sharp drop in hormone levels experienced by woman is not seen in older men [20, 21]. The most commonly experienced issue in older men is erectile dysfunction, which also increases in prevalence with ageing [21]. The exact aetiological reasons are unclear; however, disruptions in normal cell signalling due to the testosterone decrease have been identified as a potential explanatory factor. Moreover, there is some evidence that loss of mechanical sensitivity due to ageing makes erections more difficult to achieve, which may be due to natural changes in elastic and collagen fibres and smooth muscle tissue in the penis. While there is some evidence to suggest that erectile dysfunction is associated with physiological changes in ageing, these alone cannot explain the relatively high prevalence of erectile dysfunction that occurs, suggesting that its aetiology is multifaceted [21]. For more information on the prevalence of sexual dysfunction in older adults, please see Chaps. 8 and 10.

In addition to the physical factors identified, there are a number of mental health issues that can also affect the sexual health and well-being of older adults. As a person's sexuality involves the intersections of identity, expression of emotions, eroticism and fantasy, mental health and cognitive processes, the interplay between these multifaceted factors is important for sexual health in older age. Similar to physical health, older adults who enjoy good mental health are also more likely to report greater satisfaction with sexual activities. Conversely, mental health issues, such as depression and anxiety, are associated with lower levels of sexual functioning and satisfaction, with depression being the most prevalent mental health disorder in older adults [22]. Some studies reported that older men and women with depression were twice as likely to report issues with sexual health compared to those without depression [23]. For more details on mental health and sexuality in older adults, please see Chap. 4.

As people age, the size and quality of their social network changes, often reducing in size and evidencing a decline in the quality of these relationships which has an influence on the sexual lives of older adults. For example, studies indicate that amongst people over the age of 65 who have small social networks, there is a concomitant decline in levels of sexual activity and these people often report being more dissatisfied with their sex lives [22]. This finding is not surprising given that one of the most important predictors associated with sexual activity in older adults is proximity (i.e., having a sexual partner or having the possibility of finding one) [24]. Further, levels of confidence, sexual self-esteem as well as knowledge and attitudes towards their own sexuality play an important role for older adults when engaging in sexual activities. These are often influenced by societal attitudes and stigma towards sexuality of older adults, with negative stereotypes often perpetuated through the media and through medical practitioners. For more information on social issues and sexuality in older adults, please see Chaps. 12 and 13. Such issues may be even more problematic for lesbian, gay, bisexual, and transgender older adults who suffer from multiple forms of stigma related to their age as well as their sexual and/or gender identities. While little research exists in this area, some studies demonstrate that overall levels of sexual satisfaction among lesbian, gay, and bisexual older adults are lower compared to their heterosexual and/or cisgender counterparts, which may be associated with a lifetime of experiencing prejudice, discrimination, and victimization [14]. For more information on sexually and gender diverse older adults and sexual health, please see Chap. 6.

1.7 Final Note on the Book

There has long existed the need for a textbook that provides an overview of the sexuality and sexual activity in older adults. Sex and sexuality should not only be viewed from the lens of pathologies and health problems but should also be understood as a way of improving and maintaining overall health and well-being. Unfortunately, a commonality of all chapters in this book is the overall lack of evidence and research on sexuality in older adults. A common misconception is that older adults do not want to discuss sexual activities or that this topic will in a way be offensive. On the other hand enabled professionals such as healthcare workers and researchers are not trained in discussing sexual histories and lives of older adults, further contributing to this lack of information and knowledge. It is our hope that the chapters in this book will not only contain important information for practitioners and researchers but will also serve as an inspiration for further developments in the field.

References

1. World Health Organization. Ageing and health 2021 [cited 2022 27.07.2022]. https://www.who.int/news-room/fact-sheets/detail/ageing-and-health.
2. EuroStat. Healthy life years statistics 2022 [cited 2022 27.07.2022]. https://ec.europa.eu/eurostat/statistics-explained/index.php?title=Healthy_life_years_statistics.
3. Rowe JW, Kahn RL. Human aging: usual and successful. Science. 1987;237(4811):143–9. https://doi.org/10.1126/science.3299702.

4. Taylor AW. Physiology of exercise and healthy aging. Champaign, IL: Human Kinetics; 2022.
5. Clegg A, Young J, Iliffe S, Rikkert MO, Rockwood K. Frailty in elderly people. Lancet. 2013;381(9868):752–62. https://doi.org/10.1016/S0140-6736(12)62167-9.
6. Fried LP, Ferrucci L, Darer J, Williamson JD, Anderson G. Untangling the concepts of disability, frailty, and comorbidity: implications for improved targeting and care. J Gerontol A Biol Sci Med Sci. 2004;59(3):255–63. https://doi.org/10.1093/gerona/59.3.m255.
7. Manfredi G, Midao L, Paul C, Cena C, Duarte M, Costa E. Prevalence of frailty status among the European elderly population: findings from the survey of health, aging and retirement in Europe. Geriatr Gerontol Int. 2019;19(8):723–9. https://doi.org/10.1111/ggi.13689.
8. Boyd CM, Xue QL, Simpson CF, Guralnik JM, Fried LP. Frailty, hospitalization, and progression of disability in a cohort of disabled older women. Am J Med. 2005;118(11):1225–31. https://doi.org/10.1016/j.amjmed.2005.01.062.
9. Santos-Eggimann B, Karmaniola A, Seematter-Bagnoud L, Spagnoli J, Bula C, Cornuz J, et al. The Lausanne cohort Lc65+: a population-based prospective study of the manifestations, determinants and outcomes of frailty. BMC Geriatr. 2008;8:20. https://doi.org/10.1186/1471-2318-8-20.
10. Walston J, Hadley EC, Ferrucci L, Guralnik JM, Newman AB, Studenski SA, et al. Research agenda for frailty in older adults: toward a better understanding of physiology and etiology: summary from the American Geriatrics Society/National Institute on Aging research conference on frailty in older adults. J Am Geriatr Soc. 2006;54(6):991–1001. https://doi.org/10.1111/j.1532-5415.2006.00745.x.
11. Buckinx F, Rolland Y, Reginster JY, Ricour C, Petermans J, Bruyere O. Burden of frailty in the elderly population: perspectives for a public health challenge. Arch Public Health. 2015;73(1):19. https://doi.org/10.1186/s13690-015-0068-x.
12. Cruz-Jentoft AJ, Landi F, Topinkova E, Michel JP. Understanding sarcopenia as a geriatric syndrome. Curr Opin Clin Nutr Metab Care. 2010;13(1):1–7. https://doi.org/10.1097/MCO.0b013e328333c1c1.
13. Lindau ST, Gavrilova N. Sex, health, and years of sexually active life gained due to good health: evidence from two US population based cross sectional surveys of ageing. BMJ. 2010;340:c810. https://doi.org/10.1136/bmj.c810.
14. Grabovac I, Smith L, McDermott DT, Stefanac S, Yang L, Veronese N, et al. Well-being among older gay and bisexual men and women in England: a cross-sectional population study. J Am Med Dir Assoc. 2019;20(9):1080–5.e1. https://doi.org/10.1016/j.jamda.2019.01.119.
15. Lindau ST, Schumm LP, Laumann EO, Levinson W, O'Muircheartaigh CA, Waite LJ. A study of sexuality and health among older adults in the United States. N Engl J Med. 2007;357(8):762–74. https://doi.org/10.1056/NEJMoa067423.
16. Waite LJ, Laumann EO, Das A, Schumm LP. Sexuality: measures of partnerships, practices, attitudes, and problems in the National Social Life, Health, and Aging Study. J Gerontol B Psychol Sci Soc Sci. 2009;64 Suppl 1:i56–66. https://doi.org/10.1093/geronb/gbp038.
17. Salive ME. Multimorbidity in older adults. Epidemiol Rev. 2013;35:75–83. https://doi.org/10.1093/epirev/mxs009.
18. Camacho ME, Reyes-Ortiz CA. Sexual dysfunction in the elderly: age or disease? Int J Impot Res. 2005;17(Suppl 1):S52–6. https://doi.org/10.1038/sj.ijir.3901429.
19. Heidari M, Ghodusi M, Rezaei P, Kabirian Abyaneh S, Sureshjani EH, Sheikhi RA. Sexual function and factors affecting menopause: a systematic review. J Menopausal Med. 2019;25(1):15–27. https://doi.org/10.6118/jmm.2019.25.1.15.
20. Samaras N, Papadopoulou MA, Samaras D, Ongaro F. Off-label use of hormones as an antiaging strategy: a review. Clin Interv Aging. 2014;9:1175–86. https://doi.org/10.2147/CIA.S48918.
21. Seftel AD. Erectile dysfunction in the elderly: epidemiology, etiology and approaches to treatment. J Urol. 2003;169(6):1999–2007. https://doi.org/10.1097/01.ju.0000067820.86347.95.

22. Matthias RE, Lubben JE, Atchison KA, Schweitzer SO. Sexual activity and satisfaction among very old adults: results from a community-dwelling Medicare population survey. Gerontologist. 1997;37(1):6–14. https://doi.org/10.1093/geront/37.1.6.
23. Schreiner-Engel P, Schiavi RC. Lifetime psychopathology in individuals with low sexual desire. J Nerv Ment Dis. 1986;174(11):646–51. https://doi.org/10.1097/00005053-198611000-00002.
24. Smith LJ, Mulhall JP, Deveci S, Monaghan N, Reid MC. Sex after seventy: a pilot study of sexual function in older persons. J Sex Med. 2007;4(5):1247–53. https://doi.org/10.1111/j.1743-6109.2007.00568.x.

Levels and Trends of Sexual Activity in Older Adults

2

Guillermo F. López-Sánchez, José M. Oliva-Lozano, José M. Muyor, and Lee Smith

2.1 Introduction

Research in public health has found that sexual activity is associated with many aspects of life in older adults, such as well-being [1, 2], sleep quality [3], weight status [4], physical activity [5], alcohol consumption [6], smoking [7], health problems [8], chronic diseases [9], visual impairment [10], and cognitive decline [11]. However, although sexual activity can have multiple benefits and is a central component of intimate relationships, some of the studies analyzed in this chapter have reported that there tends to be a decline of sexual activity with age.

Owing to the above evidence in relation to sexual activity in older adults, it is important to know what are the levels and trends of sexual activity in this population group. Therefore, the objective of this chapter was to do a narrative review of the literature about levels and trends of sexual activity in older adults of different countries, where data allows, paying special attention to differences between countries and differences in the instruments used to measure sexual activity.

G. F. López-Sánchez (✉)
Division of Preventive Medicine and Public Health, Department of Public Health Sciences, School of Medicine, University of Murcia, Murcia, Spain
e-mail: gfls@um.es

J. M. Oliva-Lozano · J. M. Muyor
Health Research Centre, University of Almería, Almería, Spain
e-mail: jol908@ual.es; josemuyor@ual.es

L. Smith
Center for Health Performance and Wellbeing, Anglia Ruskin University, Cambridge, UK
e-mail: lee.smith@aru.ac.uk

2.2 Levels and Trends of Sexual Activity in Older Adults

In this section we analyze levels and trends of sexual activity in older adults from ten different countries: United Kingdom, United States of America, Finland, India, Cuba, Mexico, Norway, Denmark, Belgium, and Portugal.

2.2.1 United Kingdom

In a population-based study including 6201 English adults (56% women) aged 50 to >90 years [12], sexual activity decreased substantially from 50–59 years to ≥80 years in both men (from 94.1% to 31.1%) and women (from 75.9% to 14.2%). The percentage of men who reported any sexual activity in the past year was 94.1% in those aged 50–59, 84.5% in those aged 60–69 years, 59.3% in those aged 70–79 years, and 31.1% in those aged ≥80 years; in women, the respective prevalence was 75.9%, 59.9%, 34.3%, and 14.2% [12]. In other studies carried out also in English adults aged ≥50 years, the percentage of any sexual activity in the past year was 76.9–77.7% in men and 53.7–57.8% in women [1, 2].

2.2.2 United States of America

A similar trend and magnitude of decline were also observed in a US population-based study that included 3005 US adults (1550 women and 1455 men) aged 57–85 years [13]. In this study, the percentage of participants who reported any sexual activity was 73% in those aged 57–64 years, 53% in those aged 65–74 years, and 26% in those aged 75–85 years; women were significantly less likely than men at all ages to report sexual activity. This study analyzed also sexual problems by age groups, obtaining that 22–30% of men and 23–34% of women had experienced at least one sexual problem and, in consequence, they avoided sexual activity. A total of 31–45% of men indicated that they had difficulty achieving or maintaining an erection, while 36–44% of women reported difficulty with vaginal lubrication. Furthermore, 16–33% of men and 33–38% of women reported an inability to climax, and 21–30% of men declared that they climaxed too quickly [13].

2.2.3 Finland

A study carried out in Finland [14] analyzed sexual activity in 375 men and 489 women aged 55–74 years and it also observed a decline in sexual activity in the older age groups. In this study, the percentage of men who reported sexual intercourse in the last year was 87% in those aged 55–64 years and 76% in those aged 65–74 years. In the case of women, these percentages were lower: 75% in those aged 55–64 years and 48% in those aged 65–74 years. Regarding the average number of sexual partners over the lifespan, it was 18 for men of 55–64 years, nine for men of 65–74 years, and three for women of these two age groups [14].

2.2.4 India

Frequency of sexual activity was analyzed in 60 older adults (30 men and 30 women) above the age of 50 years in a study conducted in Mumbai (India) [15]. A total of 72% of participants below 60 years were sexually active, while only 57% above 60 years were active. The involvement in sexual activity by gender was also analyzed, with higher levels of sexual activity in males. A total of 40% of men and 36.7% of women reported sexual activity once per month, 36.7% of men and 6.7% of women reported sexual activity once per week, and 6.7% of men and 0% of women reported sexual activity daily [15].

2.2.5 Cuba

In Cuba, a study identified the sexual behavior in a population over 60 years of age in the health area of Tamarindo, Florencia Municipality, Ciego de Avila [16]. A total of 200 older adults (95 women and 105 men) participated in this cross-sectional descriptive study. A total of 23.2% women and 63.8% men reported to have sexual intercourse. Of those women who had sexual intercourse, the frequency of sexual activity was weekly in 18.2%, biweekly in 31.8%, and monthly in 13.6%. Of those men who had sexual intercourse, the frequency of sexual activity was weekly in 29.85%, biweekly in 37.3%, and monthly in 16.4%.

2.2.6 Mexico

A cross-sectional study was carried out in 100 older adults (63 women and 37 men) ≥60 years residing in Mexico City, Mexico [17]. In this study, 73% of the participants reported having sexual intercourse, 77% mentioned sexual activity as very important but only 40% considered it to be satisfactory [17].

2.2.7 Norway, Denmark, Belgium, and Portugal

An international study conducted in Norway, Denmark, Belgium, and Portugal evaluated the levels of sexual activity among older adults aged 60–75 years of these four countries [18]. The distribution of the sample was: Norway (676 men, 594 women), Denmark (530 men, 515 women), Belgium (318 men, 672 women), and Portugal (236 men, 273 women). The percentage of sexually active men in the past year ranged from 83% in Portugal to 91% in Norway, while the percentage of sexually active women in the past year ranged from 61% in Belgium to 78% in Denmark. Regarding frequency of sexual intercourse in the past month, men in Norway, Denmark, and Belgium (23–24%) most often reported 2–3 times per month, whereas most men in Portugal (29%) reported 1–3 times per week. However, masturbation was most commonly reported among Norwegian men (65%) and women (40%), and least commonly in Portugal (42% men and 27% women). Therefore, the authors of this study concluded that partnered sexual activity was more frequent in older adults of Southern Europe, and solitary sexual activity more frequent in older adults of Northern Europe [18].

2.3 Instruments Used to Measure Sexual Activity in Older Adults

The studies reviewed in this chapter used different questionnaires to measure sexual activity in older adults. All the questionnaires used to measure sexual activity were not validated, except the SRA-Q ELSA (Sexual Relationships and Activities Questionnaire of the English Longitudinal Study of Ageing), which is composed of items taken from validated instruments [19]. Details about this questionnaire can be found at the web of the English Longitudinal Study of Ageing [19]. Therefore, it is recommended that future studies use SRA-Q ELSA to evaluate sexual activity in older adults.

2.4 Conclusions

Considering the studies reviewed, levels of sexual activity decrease with increasing age. According to gender, sexual activity is more frequent in men than in women. These age and gender trends are similar in all the countries studied, although partnered sexual activity is more frequent in older adults of Southern Europe and solitary sexual activity more frequent in older adults of Northern Europe. Most instruments used to measure sexual activity are not validated, apart from SRA-Q ELSA.

Future research should analyze sexual activity of older adults in countries where no data is available yet, using validated instruments such as SRA-Q ELSA. Moreover, intervention programs that inform older adults about the benefits of sexual activity are recommended, and these programs should focus on those older adults of higher age, on female older adults, and on older adults from Northern Europe.

References

1. Smith L, Yang L, Veronese N, Soysal P, Stubbs B, Jackson SE. Sexual activity is associated with greater enjoyment of life in older adults. Sex Med. 2019;7(1):11–8.
2. Jackson SE, Firth J, Veronese N, Stubbs B, Koyanagi A, Yang L, Smith L. Decline in sexuality and wellbeing in older adults: a population-based study. J Affect Disord. 2019;245:912–7.
3. Smith L, Grabovac I, Veronese N, Soysal P, Isik AT, Stubbs B, Yang L, Jackson SE. Sleep quality, duration, and associated sexual function at older age: findings from the English Longitudinal Study of Ageing. J Sex Med. 2019;16(3):427–33.
4. Smith L, Yang L, Forwood S, López-Sánchez G, Koyanagi A, Veronese N, Soysal P, Grabovac I, Jackson S. Associations between sexual activity and weight status: findings from the English Longitudinal Study of Ageing. PLoS One. 2019;14(9):e0221979.

5. Smith L, Grabovac I, Yang L, Veronese N, Koyanagi A, Jackson SE. Participation in physical activity is associated with sexual activity in older English adults. Int J Environ Res Public Health. 2019;16(3):489.
6. Grabovac I, Koyanagi A, Yang L, López-Sánchez GF, McDermott D, Soysal P, Turan Isik A, Veronese N, Smith L. Prospective associations between alcohol use, binge drinking and sexual activity in older adults: The English Longitudinal Study of Ageing. Psychol Sex. 2019:1–9.
7. Jackson SE, Yang L, Veronese N, Koyanagi A, López Sánchez GF, Grabovac I, Soysal P, Smith L. Sociodemographic and behavioural correlates of lifetime number of sexual partners: findings from the English Longitudinal Study of Ageing. BMJ Sex Reprod Health. 2019;45(2):138–46.
8. Jackson SE, Yang L, Koyanagi A, Stubbs B, Veronese N, Smith L. Declines in sexual activity and function predict incident health problems in older adults: prospective findings from the English Longitudinal Study of Ageing. Arch Sex Behav. 2020;49(3):929–40.
9. Grabovac I, Smith L, Yang L, Soysal P, Veronese N, Isik AT, Forwood S, Jackson S. The relationship between chronic diseases and number of sexual partners: an exploratory analysis. BMJ Sex Reprod Health 2020; 0:1–8.
10. Smith L, Koyanagi A, Pardhan S, Grabovac I, Swami V, Soysal P, Isik A, López-Sánchez GF, McDermott D, Yang L, Jackson SE. Sexual activity in older adults with visual impairment: findings from the English Longitudinal Study of Ageing. Sex Disabil. 2019;37(4):475–87.
11. Smith L, Grabovac I, Yang L, López-Sánchez GF, Firth J, Pizzol D, McDermott D, Veronese N, Jackson SE. Sexual activity and cognitive decline in older age: a prospective cohort study. Aging Clin Exp Res. 2020;32(1):85–91.
12. Lee DM, Nazroo J, O'Connor DB, Blake M, Pendleton N. Sexual health and well-being among older men and women in England: findings from the English Longitudinal Study of Ageing. Arch Sex Behav. 2016;45(1):133–44.
13. Lindau ST, Schumm LP, Laumann EO, Levinson W, O'Muircheartaigh CA, Waite LJ. A study of sexuality and health among older adults in the United States. N Engl J Med. 2007;357(8):762–74.
14. Kontula O, Haavio-Mannila E. The impact of aging on human sexual activity and sexual desire. J Sex Res. 2009;46(1):46–56.
15. Kalra G, Subramanyam A, Pinto C. Sexuality: desire, activity and intimacy in the elderly. Indian J Psychiatry. 2011;53(4):300–6.
16. Perdomo Victoria I, Oria Cruz NL, Segredo Pérez AM, Martín LX. Sexual behaviour of older adults in the Health Area of Tamarindo, 2010. Rev Cubana Med Gen Int. 2013;29(1):8–19.
17. Guadarrama RM, Ortiz Zaragoza MC, Moreno Castillo YC, González Pedraza Avilés A. Características de la actividad sexual de los adultos mayores y su relación con su calidad de vida. Rev Esp Med Quir. 2010;15(2):72–9.
18. Træen B, Štulhofer A, Janssen E, Carvalheira AA, Hald GM, Lange T, Graham C. Sexual activity and sexual satisfaction among older adults in four European countries. Arch Sex Behav. 2019;48(3):815–29.
19. English Longitudinal Study of Ageing. https://www.elsa-project.ac.uk.

Sexual Activity and Physical Health Benefits in Older Adults

Pinar Soysal and Esin Avsar

The World Health Organization defines sexuality as: "a central aspect of being human throughout life and encompasses sex, gender identities and roles, sexual orientation, eroticism, pleasure, intimacy and reproduction. Sexuality is experienced and expressed in thoughts, fantasies, desires, beliefs, attitudes, values, behaviors, practices, roles, and relationships. While sexuality can include all of these dimensions, not all of them are always experienced or expressed. Sexuality is influenced by the interaction of biological, psychological, social, economic, political, cultural, ethical, legal, historical, religious and spiritual factors" [1]. Factors related to sexuality are an important dimension of life satisfaction in adulthood, and life satisfaction is a key indicator of successful aging. While there is no single agreed definition of successful aging, the concept is often described in terms of an absence of disease, the presence of good physical and mental health, participation in social events, and satisfaction with life. In this regard, sexual aspects of aging are an unmined, significant fact which need to be addressed.

Sexuality, sexual behavior, and intimacy are important in every phase of adult life and are an important indicator of a person's quality of life. Since the positive effects of sexuality on both mental health and physical health are well established, it has become important to understand sexual activity and functioning among the elderly and to explore this subject in people's later years of life [2]. However, in clinical practice, the sexuality and sexual activity of elderly patients is not generally an area of consideration and is rarely explored with patients by clinicians during medical examination and anamnesis, and elderly patients are reluctant to raise the

---

P. Soysal (✉)
Department of Geriatric Medicine, Faculty of Medicine, Bezmialem Vakif University, Istanbul, Turkey
e-mail: psoysal@bezmialem.edu.tr

E. Avsar
Division of Internal Medicine, Akdeniz University, Antalya, Turkey

issue themselves [3]. Personal and social beliefs and pressures, hackneyed remarks, and also neglect of sexuality in the elderly during medical education are the main reasons for this situation [3]. On the other hand, many comorbid diseases affecting both physical and mental health, the use of many drugs, and many geriatric syndromes may make it difficult for physicians to evaluate the sexual activities of the elderly. However, sexual activity can have positive effects on a range of factors as people age improving physical health and reducing early mortality in the elderly.

3.1 Effects of Physical Health on Sexual Activity

Sexual functioning varies and changes across the lifespan [2]. Desire, arousal/excitement, plateau, orgasm, and resolution/refractory period can be affected by age-related changes in the sexual response cycle occurring in both men and women. Menopause in women is associated with the most significant changes, when declined estrogen levels lead to vaginal atrophy, reduced vaginal lubrication, and diminution in sensitivity of the erogenous zones [2, 4]. In addition, decreased testosterone production in women also contributes to reduction in libido and sensitivity of erogenous zones [4]. Combined hormonal reductions can lead to decreased desire, decreased duration of sexual arousal, discomfort during vaginal intercourse due to dryness, and decreased orgasm intensity [2, 4, 5]. Gradually decreasing testosterone levels in older men are associated with decreased libido and sexual functioning, but the effect is variable and less temporally related than associations with hormone decline among women [6]. The time between sexual arousal and orgasm is prolonged. Erections require more physical stimulation to achieve and decrease in their frequency and durability. Ejaculate volume during orgasm is reduced, and the refractory period is prolonged [2].

In addition to these physiological changes, the frequency and severity of comorbid diseases, and geriatric syndromes increase as people age [7]. In a study in which 2816 outpatients admitted to a geriatric clinic were evaluated regarding their geriatric syndromes, the prevalence of polypharmacy was 54.5%, urinary incontinence 47.6%, 9.6% for malnutrition, 9.6% depression, 35.1% dementia, 21.6% recurrent falls, 33.6% sarcopenia, and frailty 28.3% [7]. In the same study, it was shown that all geriatric syndromes, except depression, are more common over the age of 80 [7]. Approximately 20% of those aged 60–69 displayed no geriatric syndromes, while it has been reported that 48% of those over the age of 80 have four or more geriatric syndromes [7]. The situation appears similar for comorbid diseases. In a study in which 448,736 elderly people were evaluated in terms of 20 comorbid diseases, such as anxiety, osteoporosis, osteoarthritis, chronic renal failure, dementia, hypertension, cancer, depression, cerebrovascular and cardiovascular diseases, 90% of the patients had at least one chronic condition [8]. The same study found that men and women showed similar overall patterns of comorbidity by age. Over 90% of both men and women had at least one comorbid condition, and more than 40%

(46.0% of men and 40.8% of women) had five or more conditions. In the oldest age group, 85 years and older, 56.2% of men and 54.7% of women had five or more comorbid conditions [8]. Therefore, several diseases, geriatric syndromes, and mental illnesses may have a huge impact on sexual desire, sexuality, and sexual functioning in elderly.

Some of the most common disorders that can adversely affect sexual functioning are cerebrovascular and cardiovascular diseases, such as heart failure, hypertension, stroke, and diabetes [9, 10]. Elderly people with these diseases may fear that their illness may worsen due to increased heart rate and respiration during sexual activity or a new attack (heart attack or stroke). Sexual activity, including arousal, erection, ejaculation, orgasm, refractory period, and dissolution, develops due to changes in the autonomic nervous system. During sexual intercourse, the cardiovascular system is stimulated by the sympathetic nervous system through signals originating from the thoracic spinal cord and transmitted to the brain [11]. In studies conducted during sexual activity in volunteers monitored in the laboratory, the highest heart rate during orgasm was found to be 140–180 per minute and the average increase in blood pressure was 80/50 mmHg. Respiratory rates and tidal volumes were measured close to values seen with moderate physical exertion [12, 13]. However, the highest energy expenditure during sexual activity does not exceed the use of oxygen compared to climbing three flights of stairs or general housework activities [9]. Therefore, clinicians should be minded to convey to patients and their partners that sexual activity is not contraindicated.

However, because of this high cardiac activity, patients with stable angina may experience chest pain during or immediately after sexual intercourse [13]. In a study of 35 patients who were followed up during sexual intercourse at home, 65% of patients complained of angina and had to stop sexual activity [13]. Appropriate medical treatment, usually with beta-blockers and in some cases with prophylactic sublingual nitrates, can prevent angina and allow a normal sexual life in these patients. The relationship between erectile dysfunction and cardiovascular disease, which severely affects sexual activity, and which is particularly common over the age of 65, has been extensively studied [10, 14–16]. Like cardiovascular disease, advanced age, hypertension, diabetes mellitus, smoking, obesity, and dyslipidemia are important risk factors for erectile dysfunction [10]. Therefore, these two diseases can be considered as different symptoms of the same systemic disorder. Based on this, it can be concluded that elderly individuals with good sexual activity have fewer comorbid diseases and their physical health is also good.

Many other medical conditions affect sexual activity. Although osteoarthritis, which is common in the elderly, does not reduce sexual desire, it can reduce pleasure during sexual activity due to joint pain and stiffness [17, 18]. Diabetes mellitus, Parkinson's disease, and chronic kidney failure can cause impotence, and depression and anxiety can negatively affect sexuality in these patients [15]. Urinary incontinence can cause fear of a loss of bladder control during sexual activity, especially in women. Approximately 50% of women with stress incontinence experience sexual dysfunction [19]. Sexual desire is not affected in patients with stroke, but sexual performance is likely to be affected (e.g., male erectile dysfunction because of physical or psychological reasons, anesthetic areas, or physical limitations due to paralysis) [19].

In neurodegenerative diseases such as dementia, not only cognitive functions, but also a loss of social and behavioral control occur and disorders increase, all of which affect sexual function [20, 21]. Although discussing sexuality with elderly patients is often neglected, it seems even more controversial to discuss this issue in the case of dementia. Data on the frequency of sexual activity in dementia patients are limited, but the results show that sexual activity continues in about a quarter of dementia patients and their partners [22]. However, as we move from being cognitive healthy to mild cognitive impairment (MCI) and from MCI to dementia, lack of interest in sex, climaxing, anxiety about ability to perform, having at least one sexual problem increases [23]. In addition, previous surgeries such as mastectomy, hysterectomy, and prostatectomy can reduce the self-confidence of the patients regarding their own sexuality [19]. The components of physical health and their possible mechanisms that can affect sexual activity are shown in Table 3.1 [19].

Table 3.1 The components of physical health and their possible mechanisms that can affect sexual activity

Comorbidities	Effect on sexual activity
Cardiovascular disease (coronary heart disease, heart failure)	Fear of bringing on another heart attack if patient resumes sexual activity Dyspnea due to the pulmonary edema Erectile dysfunction
Diabetes mellitus	Erectile dysfunction
Hypertension	Erectile dysfunction Anti-hypertensive medications, such as β-blockers
Dementia	A decrease or increase in libido Inappropriate sexual behavior due to cognitive impairment Sexual disinhibition
Stroke	Sexual desire may not be impaired, but sexual performance is likely to be affected (e.g., male erectile dysfunction because of physical or psychological reasons, anesthetic areas, or physical limitations due to paralysis)
Incontinence	Stress type incontinence can cause sexual dysfunction in women
Chronic pulmonary disease	Dyspnea during sexual activity
Chronic kidney disease	Impotence, depression, anxiety
Parkinson disease	Lack of sexual desire in men and women; impotence in men
Osteoarthritis	Disability and pain may interfere with performance
Surgery	
– Mastectomy	Emotional reactions such as depression, loss of sexual desire because of emotional reactions of patient and partner
– Hysterectomy	Depression, possible reduction in sensation during orgasm
– Prostatectomy	Impotence

3.2 Effects of Sexual Activity on Physical Health

As established, sex, and sexuality, is a key aspect of healthy adulthood. Healthy sexual activity can play a role in improving the quality of life by positively affecting emotional, mental, and physical health. With the prolongation of human life and the increase in the proportion of sexually active elderly individuals, the number of patients over the age of 65 who present to clinicians with some form of sexual dysfunction or difficulty is increasing. Perspectives, beliefs, and attitudes regarding the role that having a healthy sex life in later life is changing day by day, and medications and other treatments are being developed that enable individuals to maintain successful sexual functioning regardless of their age [2, 14]. Such treatments and interventions help facilitate continued sexual activity in participants later life.

Physical health appears to be a factor of significant influence for older men, while the quality of the relationship is the most important factor for older women [24]. Several biological mechanisms have been proposed that reveal the relationship between frequency of sexual activity and survival [19]. In a study by De Baca et al., a positive relationship between sexual intercourse and telomere length was found [25]. Telomeres are repeating nucleoprotein sequences (TTAGGG) that stabilize the ends of chromosomes and protect DNA material from duplication and degradation, which may have positive effect on sexuality [25]. Another possible mechanism could be related to the testosterone hormone levels secreted. Overall, low testosterone levels have been found to be associated with low sexual desire and higher levels of cardiovascular disease [26].

A growing literature has documented associations between engaging in sexual activity and better health and well-being outcomes [27]. Studies have shown that a higher frequency of sexual activity is associated with a number of benefits for physical health, including a reduction in cardiovascular events in later life, reduced risk of fatal coronary events, prostate and breast cancer, and better reported quality of life [28–30]. While the cross-sectional design employed by the majority of these studies means it is not clear whether sexual activity promotes good physical health or whether good physical health promotes a higher frequency of sexual activity (or indeed, whether the relationship is bidirectional), there are plausible mechanisms by which sexual activity may be beneficial for health and well-being. First, sexual activity can be considered a form of physical activity and thus those who engage in regular sexual activity likely yield the physical health benefits acquired from a physically active lifestyle [31]. Secondly, during sexual activity or at the time sexual intercourse is at its peak, there is a release of endorphins, endogenous opioid peptides that function as neurotransmitters, which generate a happy or blissful feeling [30, 32]. Circulating endorphin levels have been shown to be associated with higher natural killer cell activity which may be associated with a lower risk of cancer and viruses, and they have also been found to prevent against infections of the lungs and play an important role in improving asthma and many other conditions [33].

The most important indicator of physical health in the elderly is frailty [34]. Age-associated decline in reserve and function may result in a reduced ability to cope with acute or external stressors faced every day, which is typically defined as frailty [7, 34]. Frailty is one of the geriatric syndromes that has been subject to significant academic inquiry and scrutiny over the last two decades. Physical frailty, often termed phenotypic or syndromic frailty, was developed in part to capture representative signs and symptoms (fatigue, low activity, weakness, weight loss, and slow gait) of community-dwelling older adults that were most vulnerable to adverse health outcomes [7]. According to a meta-analysis in which 32 cross-sectional studies were included, the prevalence of frailty was 13.9%, while the prefrailty frequency was 49.4% [34]. Although there is no study showing how frailty, which as established is the most important indicator of physical health in the elderly, is affected by sexual activity, it may be considered that the factors responsible for frailty onset may be positively affected by sexual activity and that sustained sexual activity in later life may temper the onset of frailty and frailty type symptomology.

Despite the increasing interest in frailty, the underlying and preceding pathophysiological changes are not clearly known. Inflammation is one such potential pathophysiological change that may be closely linked with frailty [35]. Proinflammatory cytokines may influence frailty either directly by promoting protein degradation or indirectly by affecting important metabolic pathways [36]. A direct association between frailty and elevated levels of inflammation, as marked by elevated interleukin-6 (IL-6), C-reactive protein (CRP), fibrinogen, and factor VIII, independent of common chronic disease states has been observed [37]. Sexual activity, which is also considered as a form of physical activity, can help prevent frailty development by reducing inflammation. For example, it has been shown that inflammatory markers detected higher in ankylosing spondylitis patients compared to healthy controls may decrease with sexual function and sexual desire [38]. In another study involving 4554 elderly people, a negative correlation was found between the frequency of sexual activity and inflammatory markers (CRP, fibrinogen, and white blood cell count) [39].

Another hypothesis that is thought to cause the development of frailty is that sex hormones such as testosterone and estrogen decrease with age [40]. The most important hormone, which increases for sexual desire and during sexual activity in both women and men, is testosterone, which also has anabolic properties. Therefore, it has been shown that low testosterone levels are associated with frailty, especially in aging men [40]. A positive association of testosterone with physical performance has been reported up to a threshold of total testosterone of 15.6 nmol/L, lower free testosterone levels are associated with mobility limitation, and men with higher baseline total testosterone levels experience reduced loss of lean mass [41, 42]. In the Concord Health and Male Aging Project, low total and free testosterone were associated with frailty, and the reduction in total or free testosterone was associated with the predicted progression or increase in the severity of frailty in older men [43]. Therefore, observational data support a relationship between lower testosterone levels and increased risk of frailty in older men. Similar studies have shown the association of low testosterone levels with the development of sarcopenia in elderly women [44]. Higher levels of testosterone in those with regular sexual activity than those without sexual activity can eliminate the above-mentioned negative effects and reduce muscle loss and frailty development (Fig. 3.1).

The factors that have the most impact on both physical health and frailty are the enjoyment of life and the presence of any forms of depression and depressive symptomologies in the elderly. In numerous studies of the English Longitudinal Study of Aging working group evaluating the effects of sexual activity in the elderly it was found that among sexually active men, frequent (≥2 times a month) sexual intercourse and frequent kissing, petting, or fondling were associated with greater enjoyment of life and among sexually active women, frequent kissing, petting, or fondling was also associated with greater enjoyment of life, but there was no significant association with frequent intercourse [27]. Enjoying life is very important because enjoying life and sexual activity contributes to successful aging [45]. Palmore noted that the three strongest predictors of life satisfaction identified in the Second Duke Longitudinal Study were social activity, health, and sexual enjoyment [46]. Despite the recognition that sexual expression should be an integral part of healthy aging, research linking sexuality and successful aging is limited.

In a sample of 127 Israeli women aged ≥45 years (the majority of whom were in the 55–65 age group), Woloski-Wruble et al. explored the associations between life satisfaction and sexual activity and satisfaction with one's sex life. Although their study was conceptualized using the Rowe and Kahn model, the authors did not operationalize successful aging, but used the Life Satisfaction Index as a proxy. After reporting that life satisfaction was significantly correlated with sexual satisfaction, the authors concluded that women's satisfaction with their sex life "is an important contribution to achieving successful aging" [47]. In a similar study, Thompson et al. explored the associations among self-rated successful aging, indicators of physical and psychological health, sexual function, sexual activity, and

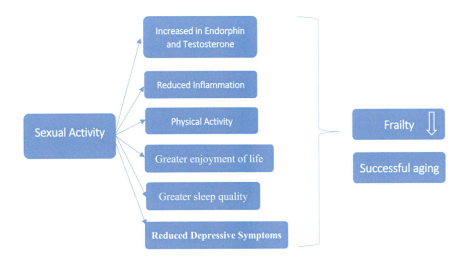

Fig. 3.1 Effects of Sexual activity on physical health

sexual satisfaction [48]. In their community-based sample of 1235 women aged 60–89 years, of whom 53% were married or in an intimate relationship, the authors found that their single-item measure of self-rated successful aging (a construct not defined in the questionnaire) was significantly correlated with sexual desire and sexual activity. Clearly, preliminary evidence suggests a relationship between sexuality and successful aging in older adults [49]. Finally, a study conducted in four European countries (Norway, Denmark, Belgium, and Portugal) showed an association between sexual activity and sexual enjoyment and successful aging in the past 10 years in both genders [45].

3.3 Conclusion

Physicians should acknowledge their personal values and attitudes regarding sex and sexuality in later life, as well as the values and attitudes of older patients. They should integrate sexual functioning (history and current) during a medical examination or treatment because medical conditions can adversely affect sexuality. Sexual problems such as erectile dysfunction can also be an early warning sign of a medical condition. Most older patients are willing to talk about their sexual concerns but are reluctant to start the discussion. They should therefore be invited by the physician, who in turn needs to be able to talk about sex freely and in a comforting manner. Older patients are usually unaware of how sexual difficulties can be related to a medical condition and are often not informed about treatment possibilities or side effects of medications. As sexual activity has extremely important and positive effects on physical health, evaluation of sexuality should be a part of geriatric evaluation. Clinicians should try to review and eliminate medical conditions that make sexual activity difficult, and inform their patients and partners about available treatment options to relieve sexual dysfunction. In fact, the frequency and continuity of sexual activity in the aging process should be kept in mind as an important step to minimize sexual dysfunction in late old age.

References

1. Gruskin S, Yadav V, Castellanos-Usigli A, Khizanishvili G, Kismödi E. Sexual health, sexual rights and sexual pleasure: meaningfully engaging the perfect triangle. Sex Reprod Health Matters. 2019;27(1):1593787. PMID: 31533569; PMCID: PMC7887957. https://doi.org/10.1080/26410397.2019.1593787.
2. Srinivasan S, Glover J, Tampi RR, Tampi DJ, Sewell DD. Sexuality and the older adult. Curr Psychiatry Rep. 2019;21:97.
3. Snyder RJ, Zweig RA. Medical and psychology students' knowledge and attitudes regarding aging and sexuality. Gerontol Geriatr Educ. 2010;31:235–55.
4. Agronin ME. Sexuality and aging. In: Steffens DC, Blazer DG, Thakur ME, editors. Textbook of geriatric psychiatry. Arlington, VA: American Psychiatric Publishing; 2015.
5. Wang V, Depp CA, Ceglowski J, Thompson WK, Rock D, Jeste DV. Sexual health and function in later life: a population-based study of 606 older adults with a partner. Am J Geriatr Psychiatry. 2015;23(3):227–33.

6. Haider A, Meergans U, Traish A, Saad F, Doros G, Lips P, et al. Progressive improvement of T-scores in men with osteoporosis and subnormal serum testosterone levels upon treatment with testosterone over six years. Int J Endocrinol. 2014;2014:496948.
7. Ates Bulut E, Soysal P, Isik AT. Frequency and coincidence of geriatric syndromes according to age groups: single-center experience in Turkey between 2013 and 2017. Clin Interv Aging. 2018;13:1899–905.
8. Gruneir A, Markle-Reid M, Fisher K, Reimer H, Ma X, Ploeg J. Comorbidity burden and health services use in community-living older adults with diabetes mellitus: a retrospective cohort study. Can J Diabetes. 2016;40(1):35–42.
9. Jaarsma T, Fridlund B, Mårtensson J. Sexual dysfunction in heart failure patients. Curr Heart Fail Rep. 2014;11(3):330–6.
10. Sooriyamoorthy T, Leslie SW. Erectile dysfunction. Treasure Island, FL: StatPearls; 2020.
11. Rampin O, Giuliano F. Central control of the cardiovascular and erection systems: possible mechanisms and interactions. Am J Cardiol. 2000;86(2A):19F–22F.
12. H Masters W, E Johnson V. Human sexual response. Boston: Little, Brown; 1966.
13. Jackson G. Sexual intercourse and angina pectoris. Br Med J. 1978;2(6129):16.
14. Valladales-Restrepo LF, Machado-Alba JE. Pharmacological treatment and inappropriate prescriptions for patients with erectile dysfunction. Int J Clin Pharmacol. 2020;43(4):900–8.
15. Pizzol D, Xiao T, Yang L, Demurtas J, McDermott D, Garolla A, et al. Prevalence of erectile dysfunction in patients with chronic kidney disease: a systematic review and meta-analysis. Int J Impot Res. 2021;33(5):508–15.
16. Pizzol D, Demurtas J, Stubbs B, Soysal P, Mason C, Isik AT, et al. Relationship between cannabis use and erectile dysfunction: a systematic review and meta-analysis. Am J Mens Health. 2019;13(6):1557988319892464.
17. Kazarian GS, Lonner JH, Hozack WJ, Woodward L, Chen AF. Improvements in sexual activity after total knee arthroplasty. J Arthroplasty. 2017;32(4):1159–63.
18. Tuominen U, Blom M, Hirvonen J, Seitsalo S, Lehto M, Paavolainen P, et al. The effect of co-morbidities on health-related quality of life in patients placed on the waiting list for total joint replacement. Health Qual Life Outcomes. 2007;5:16.
19. Hartmans CG. Sexuality in old age. In: Brocklehurst's textbook of geriatric medicine and gerontology. 8th ed. Amsterdam: Elsevier; 2016. p. 831–5.
20. Hartmans C, Comijs H, Jonker C. Cognitive functioning and its influence on sexual behavior in normal aging and dementia. Int J Geriatr Psychiatry. 2014;29(5):441–6.
21. Derouesné C, Guigot J, Chermat V, Winchester N, Lacomblez L. Sexual behavioral changes in Alzheimer disease. Alzheimer Dis Assoc Disord. 1996;10(2):86–92.
22. Ballard CG, Solis M, Gahir M, Cullen P, George S, Oyebode F, et al. Sexual relationships in married dementia sufferers. Int J Geriatr Psychiatry. 1997;12(4):447–51.
23. Lindau ST, Dale W, Feldmeth G, Gavrilova N, Langa KM, Makelarski JA, et al. Sexuality and cognitive status: a U.S. nationally representative study of home-dwelling older adults. J Am Geriatr Soc. 2018;66(10):1902–10.
24. Schick V, Herbenick D, Reece M, Sanders SA, Dodge B, Middlestadt SE, et al. Sexual behaviors, condom use, and sexual health of Americans over 50: implications for sexual health promotion for older adults. J Sex Med. 2010;7(Suppl 5):315–29.
25. Cabeza de Baca T, Epel ES, Robles TF, Coccia M, Gilbert A, Puterman E, et al. Sexual intimacy in couples is associated with longer telomere length. Psychoneuroendocrinology. 2017;81:46–51.
26. Kloner RA, Carson C 3rd, Dobs A, Kopecky S, Mohler ER 3rd. Testosterone and cardiovascular disease. J Am Coll Cardiol. 2016;67(5):545–57.
27. Smith L, Yang L, Veronese N, Soysal P, Stubbs B, Jackson SE. Sexual activity is associated with greater enjoyment of life in older adults. Sex Med. 2019;7(1):11–8.
28. Flynn T-J, Gow AJ. Examining associations between sexual behaviours and quality of life in older adults. Age Ageing. 2015;44(5):823–8.
29. Brody S, Preut R. Vaginal intercourse frequency and heart rate variability. J Sex Marital Ther. 2003;29(5):371–80.

30. Brody S, Costa RM. Sexual satisfaction and health are positively associated with penile-vaginal intercourse but not other sexual activities. Am J Public Health. 2012;102:6–7.
31. Smith L, Grabovac I, Yang L, Veronese N, Koyanagi A, Jackson SE. Participation in physical activity is associated with sexual activity in older English adults. Int J Environ Res Public Health. 2019;16(3):489.
32. Rokade P. Release of endomorphin hormone and its effects on our body and moods: a review. Int Conf Chem Biol Environ Sci. 2011;431127(215):436–8.
33. Dedenkov AN, Raĭkhlin NT, Kvetnoĭ IM, Kurilets ES, Balmasova IP. Immunohistochemical and electron microscopic identification of serotonin, melatonin and beta-endorphin in the granules of natural killers. Biull Eksp Biol Med. 1986;102(10):491–3.
34. Soysal P, Stubbs B, Lucato P, Luchini C, Solmi M, Peluso R, et al. Inflammation and frailty in the elderly: a systematic review and meta-analysis. Ageing Res Rev. 2016;31:1–8.
35. Chen X, Mao G, Leng SX. Frailty syndrome: an overview. Clin Interv Aging. 2014;9:433–41.
36. Lang P-O, Michel J-P, Zekry D. Frailty syndrome: a transitional state in a dynamic process. Gerontology. 2009;55(5):539–49.
37. Newman AB, Gottdiener JS, Mcburnie MA, Hirsch CH, Kop WJ, Tracy R, et al. Associations of subclinical cardiovascular disease with frailty. J Gerontol A Biol Sci Med Sci. 2001;56(3):M158–66.
38. Sariyildiz MA, Batmaz I, Dilek B, Inanir A, Bez Y, Tahtasiz M, et al. Relationship of the sexual functions with the clinical parameters, radiological scores and the quality of life in male patients with ankylosing spondylitis. Rheumatol Int. 2013;33(3):623–9.
39. Allen MS. Biomarkers of inflammation mediate an association between sexual activity and quality of life in older adulthood. J Sex Med. 2017;14(5):654–8.
40. Yeap BB. Hormones and health outcomes in aging men. Exp Gerontol. 2013;48(7):677–81.
41. O'Donnell AB, Travison TG, Harris SS, Tenover JL, McKinlay JB. Testosterone, dehydroepiandrosterone, and physical performance in older men: results from the Massachusetts Male Aging Study. J Clin Endocrinol Metab. 2006;91(2):425–31.
42. Krasnoff JB, Basaria S, Pencina MJ, Jasuja GK, Vasan RS, Ulloor J, et al. Free testosterone levels are associated with mobility limitation and physical performance in community-dwelling men: the Framingham Offspring Study. J Clin Endocrinol Metab. 2010;95(6):2790–9.
43. Travison TG, Nguyen A-H, Naganathan V, Stanaway FF, Blyth FM, Cumming RG, et al. Changes in reproductive hormone concentrations predict the prevalence and progression of the frailty syndrome in older men: the concord health and ageing in men project. J Clin Endocrinol Metab. 2011;96(8):2464–74.
44. Yuki A, Ando F, Otsuka R, Shimokata H. Low free testosterone is associated with loss of appendicular muscle mass in Japanese community-dwelling women. Geriatr Gerontol Int. 2015;15(3):326–33.
45. Štulhofer A, Hinchliff S, Jurin T, Hald GM, Træen B. Successful aging and changes in sexual interest and enjoyment among older European men and women. J Sex Med. 2018;15(10):1393–402.
46. Palmore E. Predictors of successful aging. Gerontologist. 1979;19(5 Pt 1):427–31.
47. Woloski-Wruble AC, Oliel Y, Leefsma M, Hochner-Celnikier D. Sexual activities, sexual and life satisfaction, and successful aging in women. J Sex Med. 2010;7(7):2401–10.
48. Thompson WK, Charo L, Vahia IV, Depp C, Allison M, Jeste DV. Association between higher levels of sexual function, activity, and satisfaction and self-rated successful aging in older postmenopausal women. J Am Geriatr Soc. 2011;59(8):1503–8.
49. Kleinstäuber M. Factors associated with sexual health and well being in older adulthood. Curr Opin Psychiatry. 2017;30(5):358–68.

Sexual Activity and Mental Health Benefits in Older Adults

4

Tobias Schiffler, Hanna M. Mües, and Igor Grabovac

Both the relative and absolute proportion of older persons in the global population are rapidly increasing [1]. Especially countries in Europe, Asia, North and South America are anticipated to be primarily affected by this trend and will have a proportion of the population aged 60 years or older of above 30% by 2050. In this regard, the global population of people over 60 years of age will almost double with an estimated rise from 12% to 22% [2]. Additionally, the general pace of population aging also increased dramatically. This development is caused by two key drivers, namely growing life expectancy and a decrease in fertility rates globally [1].

4.1 The Relationship Between Aging and Sexuality

The process of aging can be described in several ways. From a biological point of view, it is characterized as a lifelong and gradual accumulation of cellular and molecular damage that leads to impairment in various bodily functions and contributes to a general vulnerability and an increase in risk of mortality and morbidity [1]. Beyond that, aging can also be viewed both from a psychological and a social perspective, which can be influenced by the biological changes. As aging is characterized by progressive metabolic and biochemical changes, these may exert an influence on mood, attitudes toward the environment, physical condition, and social activity [3]. This transition subsequently causes a change in the positions of older

---

T. Schiffler · I. Grabovac (✉)
Department of Social and Preventive Medicine, Center for Public Health, Medical University of Vienna, Vienna, Austria
e-mail: tobias.schiffler@meduniwien.ac.at; igor.grabovac@meduniwien.ac.at

H. M. Mües
Department of Clinical and Health Psychology, Faculty of Psychology, University of Vienna, Vienna, Austria
e-mail: hanna.mues@univie.ac.at

© Springer Nature Switzerland AG 2023
L. Smith, I. Grabovac (eds.), *Sexual Behaviour and Health in Older Adults*, Practical Issues in Geriatrics, https://doi.org/10.1007/978-3-031-21029-7_4

people within the family and society. The extent to which persons of advanced age respond to these changes depends on their awareness and adaptability to the aging process. From a psychological perspective, advancing age can often cause problems in adapting to new situations as well as unfavorable changes on a cognitive level. In terms of social aspects, the process of aging can affect an individual's position within the community. While these complex processes require a high degree of self-control and self-regulation on the part of older people, inadequate attempts at adaptation can be accompanied by deficits, which can subsequently have a negative impact on the quality of life of those affected. Eventually, these effects represent risk factors for impaired mental health. In terms of a personal life of high quality and meaningfulness, sexuality is considered pivotal [4]. Relating to the term "sexuality," it is described as the ability to experience sexual feelings and includes a variety of aspects, among which are gender identity, eroticism, intimacy, sexual orientation, and social aspects of sex [5]. In a broader context, sexuality can be viewed as a dynamic outcome of attitudes, motivation, physical capacity, opportunity for partnership, and sexual conduct [6]. Also, it should be mentioned that sexuality is not merely the act of sexual intercourse but may also comprise touching, caressing, fantasy, masturbation, physical closeness, and warmth arising from shared emotionality between human beings. Regarding quality of life, sexuality and intimacy are essential contributing factors and maintain meaningfulness over a person's entire lifespan. It must therefore be taken into account that sexuality is an important dimension of life satisfaction, where it is important in terms of expressing love and caring. This aspect is especially important for people of older age [7, 8]. Particularly in late adulthood sexual activity is vital on many levels. Not only is sexuality an expression of passion or affection, but also signals loyalty, trust, and mutual admiration. Beyond that, sexual activity is highly relevant for older adults in order to maintain higher energy levels, enhance their self-confidence, and further develop their capability to comply with their needs and wants [8]. It is a way to affirm physical ability and can therefore be seen as a mechanism to cope with the aging process. Moreover, a number of publications indicated that sexual inactivity is associated with poor health conditions, such as hypertension, diabetes, and cardiovascular problems [9, 10]. A similar relationship can be seen between sexual inactivity and mental health, as the lack of sexual activity has been linked to a variety of problematic mental health outcomes, such as depression or poor self-reported quality of life [11].

4.2　Mental Health and Social Aspects of Sexuality in Older Adults

Sexual health refers to a constitutive part of reproductive health, which is defined as peoples' ability to have a satisfying, responsible, and safe sex life [12]. Sexuality and mental health are linked in many ways. In particular, there is an association between mental health and overall sexual satisfaction. A range of mood, anxiety, and substance use disorders have been shown to be related with general sexual dissatisfaction, while this link is independent of sociodemographic and experiential factors [13]. It is therefore important to keep in mind that people living with mental disorders are susceptible to experience further deficits in their mental well-being, as proper sexual functioning is a constitutive component of quality of life and maintaining satisfying intimate relationships [14]. Mental health and the social environment of individuals appear to be determinants for the frequency of a person's sexual activities [15, 16]. Based on data from the United States of America and the United Kingdom, many older adults have intimate relationships and consider sexuality as an important part of life that contributes to an overall emotional well-being. Although sexual activity and sexual fulfillment are ubiquitous parts of human life, stereotypes regarding the elderly typically ignore their significance for this population [17]. However, both the quality and quantity of sexual activities are highly important factors for the mental health of older adults [18]. In this respect, better mental health among older persons is associated with feeling satisfied with sexual activities and their frequency. Furthermore, it increases an individual's satisfaction with their sexual life, which is defined as the subjectively perceived quality of sexuality, sexual life, and sexual relationships and also refers to a person's sexual well-being [19]. Also, the effects of sex on mental health can partially be explained by the quality of the relationship to the sexual partner. Not only exogenous but also endogenous factors exhibit an association between sexual activity and mental health. For example, sexual activities usually foster relaxation, social attachment, and a feelings of love, which lead to a release of dopamine, endorphins, and oxytocin causing a reduction in anxiety and stress [20]. Furthermore, subjective assessment of sexual activity can be seen as a determinant of mental health, especially for older persons who experienced a decrease in the frequency of sexual activities, whereby both the excess and deprivation of sexual activities in comparison to the actual want of an individual are highly related with low interpersonal relationship quality and low mental health outcomes [18, 21]. As the impact of sexual activity is not solely limited to mental health outcomes it should also be taken into account that on a physical level poor sexual activity shows an association with cardiovascular risk factors and conditions such as hypertension, cancer, high cholesterol, and diabetes for both women and men [22–24]. Regarding physical outcomes, major surgery as well as conditions inducing pain, compromising mobility or energy reserve, or those directly interfering with partnered sex are also related to reduced sexual activity [11]. In terms of mental health, considering chronic physical outcomes is essential as mental health and physical health are fundamentally linked. Individuals living with chronic physical health issues experience depression and anxiety twice as often compared to the general population [25]. In further consequence these mental health issues can lead to an impairment of a person's sexuality and sexual activity, which can additionally contribute to a reduction of emotional, psychological, and social well-being.

Good sexual health does not merely imply the absence of impairment, dysfunction, or disease, but also premises an affirmative approach to sexuality. Moreover, sexual relationships as well as the possibility of having enjoyable and safe sexual experiences are essential components of sexual health. These sexual experiences must be free of coercion, discrimination, and violence. The sexual rights of an individual have to be approached in a respectful, protective, and fulfilling way, in order to lead to good sexual health. Particularly as in the past, the issue of sexual health was viewed almost solely in terms of the possible negative consequences for physical and mental health [26], with attention being primarily focused on sexually transmitted diseases, unplanned pregnancy, sexual dysfunction, sexual assault, and sexual violence. However, a new discourse has developed in various disciplines concerning sexual health issues that focuses more on the positive aspects of sexuality. Sexual, physical, and mental health, as well as overall well-being are positively associated with sexual self-esteem, sexual pleasure, and sexual satisfaction [27, 28]. The positive effects of sexual satisfaction should be addressed in programs that aim to improve these health outcomes. For that purpose, service delivery, prevention, and sexual education should be taken into account.

Evidence of the association between mental health and sexual health has been researched both in the general adult population and in older adults particularly [29]. This could potentially be due to the fact that an increasing number of older women and men experience the age period of 60–75 as a rather energetic and healthy time of their lives [30]. Furthermore, older adults who are sexually active show a higher frequency of petting, kissing, and fondling, which is associated with a higher enjoyment of life [31]. In comparison with sexually inactive older adults, those who report higher sexual activity levels also report having higher scores for sexual and global life satisfaction [19, 32, 33]. These findings can be set against the general stereotypes of asexuality in older adulthood, as an increasing number of people remain sexually active in later life [17]. This progression can be explained by several trends; first, there is a general increase in life expectancy and people reach the older age in better health, and secondly, social attitudes toward sex in later life are slowly shifting toward a wider recognition within society. More than ever is sexual expression recognized as an integral part of human life in terms of maintaining interpersonal relationships, the promotion of self-esteem, and the contribution to health and well-being even in older adults [34, 35]. In this context, sexual expression is an umbrella term for sexual behavior, sexual desire, wanted sexual behavior, arousal, and lust [36]. However, evidence shows that sexual expression changes during the course of life and with rising age as previously outlined in terms of activities and frequency [34].

The asexual stereotype of older adulthood is prominent within the general population, where it is predominantly manifested in negative reactions and emotions, such as embarrassment, shame, and disgust against older persons' sexual expression [37]. Many theories exist that try to explain how these stereotypes develop and where they are established. In this respect, among the most elaborated theories, there are two developmental theories which are based on evolution and disengagement [38]. Evolutionary theory postulates that the act of sexual intercourse pursues a merely functional purpose, which aims at procreation. Based on this theory, older adults are not to be seen as fertile individuals and are therefore asexual beings. As another developmental theory, the disengagement theory suggests that individuals and whole societies reciprocally withdraw from each other in later life [39]. This theory leads on to a reinforcement of ageism by theorizing that people of advanced age consciously conduct a shift of their interaction style from active to passive. According to this theory, asexuality occurs subsequently to social passivity.

Due to the aforementioned assumptions on asexuality in older adults, the research interest for this field has been underdeveloped and largely ignored by both the academic and clinical establishments. Only in the last few decades, with growing focus on health and active aging and developments in the field of gerontology and geriatrics and various pharmaceutical and technological advancements, have these topics been placed under somewhat larger focus [40]. However the preconceived notions are still largely dominant, even as several studies have outlined that many older individuals remain sexually active even in older age [23, 41, 42], even as activities move away from penetrative sex toward other types of activities such as masturbation, petting, and fondling [30]. For older adults who also report not engaging actively in sexual activities, sexuality still remains an important part of their lives as sexuality and sexual desire remain vital components of close emotional relationships in later life [37, 43]. Older adults also view sexual activities as a source of vitality and youthfulness, a way of staying emotionally connected to their partners, and a way to experience pleasure [44]. Some of the benefits of sexual activity on mental health in older adults based on the available literature are listed in Table 4.1.

Table 4.1 Benefits of sexuality on mental health of older adults

1	Sexual intercourse with one's partner leads to a closer relationship between individuals, and closeness to a partner is associated with well-being
2	Emotional closeness between partnered persons during sexual intercourse is beneficial to a higher enjoyment of life
3	More frequent kissing, petting, and fondling are associated with greater life enjoyment
4	Sexual activity is beneficial to a person's general health, which affects life satisfaction in a positive way
5	As the body releases endorphins during sexual activity or orgasms, a happy or blissful feeling is generated subsequently
6	As physical activity per se shows beneficial effects on a person's mental health, and sexual intercourse is a form of physical activity, it contributes to an improvement of psychological aspects
7	Concerns about the sex life of older adults are negatively associated with life enjoyment, which is why a reduction of these concerns could lead to a higher quality of life. In this regard, an additional relation to the advantages of an active and problem-free sex life seems to be likely
8	Sexual activity in older adults is an adequate measure to prevent mental health complications, such as depression and anxiety, which is why other measures should focus on maintaining sexuality
9	Especially for men, a higher frequency of sexual intercourse is associated with greater life enjoyment, whereas life enjoyment of women shows a higher association with other sexual activities
10	Physical tenderness is an essential contributor to women's mental health
11	Older adults whose sexual activity is on a higher level possess more positive aging parameters and fewer chronic conditions, which leads to a greater enjoyment of life, as a consequence

4.3 Sexual Orientation, Gender Identity and Its Influence on Mental Health in Older Adulthood

People whose sexual orientation and sexual identity diverge from the heteronormative conception have had and still have to deal with a variety of barriers and discrimination. Homosexuality has been associated with illness, sin, and immorality, and is considered illicit and punishable in many countries around the world even today [45–47]. These negative experiences are also shared by people with transgender identities as they are also confronted with strong negative societal attitudes, discrimination, and a lack of understanding within their social environments [48, 49]. In this regard, older persons who are lesbian, gay, bisexual, transgender, intersexual, queer, and other minority gender identities and sexualities (LGBTIQ+) are in an especially precarious position, as they have usually been exposed to these negative experiences for longer periods of time [50]. In respect to the rapid global increase of aging populations, service providers and policy makers have to adapt to changing health and social care needs, which is why these needs, as well as their economic implications, have to be identified in order to be able to adequately respond to them [51]. In the United States of America, the number of LGBTIQ+ people above the age of 50 years is estimated to be approximately 2.4 million, and is predicted to elevate up to five million people until the year 2030 [52].

As a consequence of the negative societal attitudes, many LGBTIQ+ older individuals have been confronted with discrimination, heterosexism, homophobia, transphobia, and stigmatization during their lifetime [53]. These negativities lead to a number of other issues, such as social exclusion and worsening of physical and mental health [54, 55]. Moreover, due to the high levels of discrimination and hostility in some communities, some LGBTIQ+ older adults may be forced into cisnormativity, heteronormativity, and compulsory heterosexuality, which is further associated with a rise of discrimination and marginalization, disempowerment, and oppression, and can therefore compromise social well-being and mental health [56–58]. Many LGBTIQ+ individuals have accommodated themselves to this heteronormativity and cisnormativity, and adapted to societal prejudices. Based on this adjustment, a tension between needs and experiences is developed that may cause sexual minority stress [59]. Existing evidence shows that minority stress in general is related to mental health problems, emotional distress, and high-risk sexual behaviors, which can have significant implications for available support services for this population [60]. As a consequence of these societal issues, many LGBTIQ+ people experience further negative effects on their mental health. As studies have shown, the majority of LGBTIQ+ persons tend to be single, living alone, and childless [61, 62], with more than half reporting loneliness and isolation. It must be kept in mind that these aspects are very likely to have a negative impact on the subjective well-being and mental health of the people concerned. As opposed to this, other studies identified better self-reported well-being among individuals who have strengthening relationships [63]. LGBTIQ+ people face discrimination, rejection, prejudice, and stereotyping in many cases. This circumstance often results in these individuals feeling exposed to hostile social environments for a lifetime, while this exposure is linked to depression and low quality of life [64]. In this regard, it is particularly important for healthcare professionals to recognize signs of distress among those affected and respond to them in an adequate manner, as a positive view of one's sexual and gender identity is associated with better mental health and higher quality of life [65, 66].

In order to be able to adequately work with this population in a professional healthcare setting, it is mandatory to recognize the lived experiences and needs of LGBTIQ+ older adults. Professionals must identify strategies to facilitate access to community resources and healthcare facilities. Also, general social support networks and those specified to LGBTIQ+ persons have to be regarded as these are highly relevant in terms of mental and physical health and possess a potential to influence those individuals in a strongly positive way [62, 67]. Healthcare professionals who work in the field of gerontology must recognize that some older LGBTIQ+ persons may experience a so-called triple stigma [60], the three components being: (1) older age, which is also known as ageism; (2) prejudice regarding the gender identity and sexual orientation of LGBTIQ+ people; and (3) issues associated with poor health conditions, such as mental illness, substance misuse, hepatitis, and HIV/AIDS [68]. This triple stigma further contributes to a higher risk of mental illness, isolation, and fragmentation of social networks and support. Given the impact of stigma on mental health, it is highly important to bear this in mind when it comes to the assessment of risk factors [69]. In order to be able to fully understand the well-being and life satisfaction of LGBTIQ+ individuals, considerations regarding intersectional backgrounds as well as age and gender identities have to be made. Especially, the conduction of programs and development of policies are dependent on these considerations, in order to specifically target this group of persons and support their mental health [70].

4.4 A Professional Approach to Sexuality in Older Adults

Considering all above-mentioned issues, all older adults are a highly vulnerable group whose needs have to be met by healthcare professionals in an adequate way. As depicted before, mental health, quality of life, and well-being are strongly associated with sexuality, sexual health, and the expression of sexual identity, which are important for the lives of older adults [37, 71]. Even as there are a number of articles and literature on the overall importance of sexuality in older adults and its benefits on mental health, this topic is still under-researched and there is a paucity of strong evidence. Healthcare professionals play a major role as gatekeepers, but frequently oversee the significance of sexual activity in people above the age of 65 [72]. Based upon available literature, healthcare professionals from different disciplines and settings generally have little knowledge of sexuality in older adults and are therefore largely unable to address this matter appropriately [73]. In a systematic review of quantitative and qualitative evidence, Bauer et al. [73] synthesized five key elements out of their findings that summarize the main aspects of older adults' recognition of sexuality in the context of healthcare settings (Table 4.2).

Table 4.2 Older adults' recognition of sexuality in healthcare settings [73]

1	Regarding the well-being of older adults, sexuality is a key component
2	When discussing sexuality in a professional healthcare setting, older people tend to use euphemistic language and assign a distinct connotation to certain terms
3	When sexuality is displayed in healthcare settings, older adults assume discretion
4	Due to the negative perceptions of older adults regarding the interest and attitudes of healthcare professionals toward sexuality and sexual health, they feel reluctant and uncomfortable coming up with these issues
5	Instead of communicating with a healthcare professional, older adults tend to experience a sexual problem in isolation, since it is common for them to be unknowing of their personal sexual health

Regarding sexuality in older adults, it is essential for healthcare professionals to approach this in a way in which patients feel understood and concerned, and are encountered with interest and empathy [74]. In order to accomplish this, professionals have to acquire a certain set of effective communication skills, especially regarding sexuality and sexual health, as current evidence shows insufficient communication between older adults and healthcare professionals in these matters, although older persons affected may have the desire to express certain concerns, and have a wish for the consultation of physicians and other health experts [75]. Nevertheless, these issues must be approached in a careful way since the privacy of people has to be respected.

For a number of reasons, many people in older adulthood experience difficulties initiating a conversation about sexuality. For this reason, they have to be actively provided the opportunity to discuss their issues and concerns by healthcare professionals in a way that feels adequate to them, and does not raise negative emotions. Due to this sensitivity, professionals working in the healthcare setting are to adopt the needful role of a facilitator through an increased awareness for the desires of older adults [76]. In order to be able to fulfill this meaningful role, healthcare professionals are required to possess a certain level of reflectivity, and are supposed to perform continuous monitoring of their personal comfort when it comes to discussing sexual health and sexuality. An essential aspect concerning this matter is their preparedness to raise these issues during sessions of consultation and their ability to provide specific care for older individuals [73].

The identification of actual needs of older persons that should lead on to positive outcomes is a main task of healthcare professionals. Raised attention to sexual activity among older adults is important in order to be able to efficiently support those individuals by identifying and properly addressing their actual needs. If this is conducted in a way that is suitable for older adults, these individuals are empowered to deal with their own sexuality and sexual health, which further contributes to an improved state of mental health. Especially, due to the fact that in some cases older people do not consider sexuality important, it is indispensable for healthcare professionals to close the gap within sensitization and training [77]. Sensitization and training should focus on the implementation of specific interventions that target the promotion of sexual activity in older aged individuals. Since this particular field includes several aspects that need to be considered, Silva et al. [77] postulated certain guiding principles for this type of interventions in the course of a qualitative research work that investigated the opinions of nurses who were experts in the context of clinical practice and teaching (Table 4.3).

As sexuality must be seen as an essential aspect in terms of active aging, healthcare professionals are encouraged to proactively address this topic with their older aged patients. This proactivity may sometimes be necessary as some older adults may feel too ashamed or shy to actively seek help by themselves, which could be accounted for by a feeling of ridiculousness that leads on to a form of resignation [78]. Offering the opportunity for an esteeming talk about sexual activity within the process of aging could act as a supportive measure for older persons, since these frequently report a lack of information and open discussion around this issue, where healthcare professionals play a particular role [79].

People of advanced ages consider their sexuality and the manifestation of their sexuality as essential components for a high quality of life. Healthcare professionals are to handle issues related to sexuality in older ages in a sensitive way, as some older people prefer to keep their sexuality completely private, and others experience a distinct desire to discuss certain aspects of their sex life and their perception of it [73]. However, this desire can be eliminated if healthcare professionals show disinterest for their patients or their thoughts and feelings, as well as negative attitudes, shame, and embarrassment. In this regard, strategies should be implemented that

Table 4.3 Guiding principles for interventions on sexuality in older adults

1	Interventions for the improvement of awareness and sensitization at the level of health promotion and disease prevention should focus on • Raising awareness about the physical, psychological, and social changes of aging, and • Achieving sensitization regarding typical characteristics of sexuality in older age and the influence of the aging process
2	Interventions should comprise defined priorities and contexts for them to be as efficient as possible
3	Interventions in the field of information should consider the concept of informotherapy, which implicates that information is given at the right dosage for the right person and at the right time
4	Interventions should aim at the identification of main barriers to sexuality, conditions that exacerbate sexual behaviors, drugs that hinder or help, myths, beliefs, and experiences of intimacy
5	Interventions aiming at the promotion of sexual health in the course of the aging process should approach this issue in a positive and respectful way
6	Interventions should promote safe and pleasant sexual experiences, free of coercion, discrimination, and violence, as this leads to an overall better mental health
7	Interventions should comprise different strategies with special adaptions for individuals, couples, groups, and communities at large
8	Interventions should integrate screenings of certain diseases and dysfunctions, as this could identify a need for sex therapy or other therapeutical interventions
9	Interventions that are related to counseling should focus on the level of permission, information, and suggestions, and should include discussing issues of sexuality
10	In order to elicit the outcome of a certain intervention, it is necessary to determine the indicators that are intended to be measured in advance

An adaption and extension of Silva et al. [77]

contribute to a safe environment in which older adults can speak about their sexuality and feel empowered. If this kind of setting is maintained, professionals and older adults can come together and discuss relevant issues regarding sexuality, because this may lead on to a situation in which older people feel enabled to be sexually active, which would further have a beneficial impact on their overall mental health, subjective quality of life, and life satisfaction.

4.5 Psychotropic Drugs and Their Negative Effects on Sexual Function

Healthcare professionals should be aware of the fact that not only mental disorders but also the psychotropic drugs used to treat them often have negative consequences on sexual desire. Sexual dysfunction (SD) is a common side effect of many psychotropic drugs. A multitude of studies report a prevalence between 60 and 80% with certain antidepressants, as well as SSRIs and up to 60% risk on SD with the use of specific antipsychotics [80–82]. However, it is difficult to make an accurate statement because the issue of sexual dysfunction in connection to psychotropic medication is characterized by high underreporting [83–85]. The importance of targeted inquiry using SD questionnaires is often emphasized to reduce this underreporting [83, 86]. The danger of not reporting is that high noncompliance can occur unnoticed, making the actual treatment less effective [86, 87].

The etiology of SD depends on several factors, as the extent to which SD is also influenced by mental illness and other factors must be considered [82]. Indeed, regardless of medication use, 50–70% of depressed patients also experience reduced interest in sexual activity [86]. Thus, the studying of its etiology is challenging. Moreover, many clinical case studies are difficult to compare, due to different methodology, diverse clinical pictures, and individual patient characteristics. In addition, the clinical picture of SD describes a broad spectrum of different complaints, starting with decreases in libido, problems with arousal and erectile dysfunction up to changes in orgasm and ejaculation disorders, issues with vaginal lubrication, painful intercourse among others. These different symptoms are sometimes based on different mechanisms and can be treated differently, which is why the comparability of groups is made even more difficult [87–89].

Through this, there are few well-done, evidence-based meta-analyses that can compare specific medications and identify which medications have the highest, or lowest, incidence of sexual side-effects. However, clear trends are evident, with the highest prevalence of SD consistently reported with serotonin-enhancing medications. Here, a 60–80% risk of SD is spoken of with the use of certain selective serotonin reuptake inhibitors (SSRIs) [80, 81].

The mechanisms of action for SD caused by antidepressants are thought to be based on the inhibitory effects of serotonin in the sexual cycle, such as inhibition of libido and orgasm, which is why the risk of sexual side effects is particularly high with SSRIs and selective norepinephrine reuptake inhibitors [90]. With regard to antipsychotics, sexual side effects occur primarily with the so-called classic/first-generation antipsychotics. Here, the mechanism of action is mainly due to the increase of prolactin, which can lead to SD [91, 92]. For antipsychotic-induced SD, there is a reported incidence of approximately 16–27% for prolactin-independent antipsychotics as well as quetiapine, ziprasidone, perphenazine, and aripiprazole, and a 40–60% risk of SD for prolactin-increasing antipsychotics, e.g., olanzapine, risperidone, haloperidol, clozapine, and thioridazine [82].

The treatment of psychotropic drugs-induced sexual dysfunction is highly individualized and determined by different factors and approaches. Again, there is little evidence-based knowledge and it is recommended to choose a treatment individually with regard to the patient's preferences [85, 86]. Treatment options include adjusting the dose, switching the medication, augmentation by adding, for example, phosphodiesterase type five inhibitors, such as sildenafil, or bupropion to the therapy, and a wide range of psychoeducational accompanying measures [85, 93, 94]. Some randomized controlled trials suggest a positive effect on sexual satisfaction from augmentation or switching to aripiprazole, or from adding mirtazapine to treatment [93, 95, 96]. Briefly interrupting SSRI use in the form of a "drug holiday" appears to work in some cases, but is controversial due to risks for withdrawal symptoms and should be further explored [93, 97].

Table 4.4 provides an overview of current psychotropic drugs and their specific sexual side effects.

Table 4.4 Psychotropic drugs and sexual side effects

Agent	Sexual side effect
Antidepressants	
SSRIs	
Citalopram	*Common:* – Loss of libido – Ejaculation disorders – Erectile dysfunction
Escitalopram	*Common:* – Decreased libido – Women: Anorgasmia – Men: Ejaculation disorders, impotence
Fluoxetine	*Common:* – Loss of libido – Ejaculation disorders – Sexual dysfunction *Uncommon:* – Abnormal orgasm – Anorgasmia
Fluvoxamine	*Uncommon:* – Delayed ejaculation
Paroxetine	*Very common:* – Sexual dysfunction

(continued)

Table 4.4 (continued)

Agent	Sexual side effect
Sertraline	*Very common:* – Ejaculatory failure *Common:* – Loss of libido – Erectile dysfunction *Rare:* – Premature ejaculation
SNRIs	
Duloxetine	*Common:* – Decreased libido – Abnormal orgasm – Erectile dysfunction – Ejaculation disorders *Uncommon:* – Sexual dysfunction
Venlafaxine	*Common:* – Decreased libido – Abnormal ejaculation/orgasm – Anorgasmia – Erectile dysfunction
TZAs	
Amitriptyline	*Common:* – Loss of libido – Impotence
Clomipramine	*Very common:* – Libido and potency disorders *Unknown frequency:* – Delayed ejaculation
Doxepin	*Unknown frequency:* – Sexual dysfunction
Nortriptyline	*Common:* – Libido and erectile dysfunction
Trimipramine	*Unknown frequency:* – Sexual dysfunction
Other antidepressants	
Agomelatine	Unreported
Bupropion	Unreported
Mirtazapine	Unreported
Moclobemide	Unreported
Tranylcypromine	*Rare:* – Anorgasmia – Erectile dysfunction – Abnormal ejaculation
Trazodone	*Uncommon:* – Erectile dysfunction
Antipsychotics	
First-generation antipsychotics	
Haloperidol	*Common:* – Erectile dysfunction *Uncommon:* – Loss of libido *Rare:* – Sexual dysfunction

Table 4.4 (continued)

Agent	Sexual side effect
Perphenazine	*Common:* – Sexual dysfunction
Pimozide	*Common:* – Erectile dysfunction *Unknown frequency:* – Decreased libido
Zuclopenthixol	*Common:* – Decreased libido – Erectile dysfunction *Uncommon:* – Increased libido – Women: Orgasm disorder – Vulvovaginal dryness
Atypical antipsychotics	
Aripiprazole	*Common ("Maintena" only):* – Erectile dysfunction *Uncommon ("Maintena" only):* – Decreased libido – Vulvovaginal dryness
Clozapine	*Unknown frequency:* – Retrograde ejaculation
Olanzapine	Unreported
Quetiapine	*Uncommon:* – Sexual dysfunction
Risperidone	*Uncommon:* – Decreased libido – Erectile dysfunction – Ejaculation disorders – Sexual dysfunction *Rare:* – Anorgasmia
Other psychotropic drugs	
Antiepileptic/anticonvulsive drugs and mood stabilizers	
Carbamazepine	*Very rare:* – Sexual dysfunction – Decreased libido – Erectile dysfunction – Decreased male fertility and/or abnormal spermatogenesis (decreased sperm count and/or motility)
Gabapentin	*Common:* – Impotence *Unknown frequency:* – Sexual dysfunction – Libido changes – Ejaculatory dysfunction – Anorgasmia
Lamotrigine	Unreported
Lithium	*Unknown frequency:* – Sexual dysfunction
Phenytoin	Unreported

(continued)

Table 4.4 (continued)

Agent	Sexual side effect
Pregabalin	*Common:* – Loss of libido – Erectile dysfunction *Uncommon:* – Increased libido – Sexual dysfunction – Delayed ejaculation
Topiramate	*Uncommon:* – Erectile dysfunction – Sexual dysfunction
Valproic acid	Unreported
Benzodiazepines	
Clonazepam	*Unknown frequency:* – Loss of libido – Erectile dysfunction
Lorazepam	*Uncommon:* – Impotence – Decreased orgasm

SNRI selective norepinephrine reuptake inhibitor, *SSRI* selective serotonin reuptake inhibitor, *TZA* tetracyclic antidepressant
Common: 1–10%; Uncommon: 0.1–1%; Rare: 0.01–0.1%; Very rare: 0.001–0.01%

References

1. World Health Organization. World report on ageing and health. Geneva: WHO Press; 2015.
2. World Health Organization. Ageing and health. 2021. https://www.who.int/news-room/fact-sheets/detail/ageing-and-health.
3. Dziechciaż M, Filip R. Biological psychological and social determinants of old age: bio-psycho-social aspects of human aging. Ann Agric Environ Med. 2014;21(4):835–8. https://doi.org/10.5604/12321966.1129943.
4. Gewirtz-Meydan A, Hafford-Letchfield T, Benyamini Y, Phelan A, Jackson J, Ayalon L. Ageism and sexuality. In: Ayalon L, Tesch-Römer C, editors. International perspectives on aging. Contemporary perspectives on ageism, vol. 19. Berlin: Springer International; 2018. p. 149–62. https://doi.org/10.1007/978-3-319-73820-8_10.
5. Dhingra I, de Sousa A, Sonavane S. Sexuality in older adults: clinical and psychosocial dilemmas. J Geriatr Mental Health. 2016;3(2):131. https://doi.org/10.4103/2348-9995.195629.
6. Ni Lochlainn M, Kenny RA. Sexual activity and aging. J Am Med Dir Assoc. 2013;14(8):565–72. https://doi.org/10.1016/j.jamda.2013.01.022.
7. Campbell JM, Huff MS. Sexuality in the older woman. Gerontol Geriatr Educ. 1996;16(1):71–81. https://doi.org/10.1300/J021v16n01_07.
8. Skałacka K, Gerymski R. Sexual activity and life satisfaction in older adults. Psychogeriatrics. 2019;19(3):195–201. https://doi.org/10.1111/psyg.12381.
9. Friedman S. Cardiac disease, anxiety, and sexual functioning. Am J Cardiol. 2000;86(2):46–50. https://doi.org/10.1016/s0002-9149(00)00893-6.
10. Miner M, Esposito K, Guay A, Montorsi P, Goldstein I. Cardiometabolic risk and female sexual health: the Princeton III summary. J Sex Med. 2012;9(3):641–51; quiz 652. https://doi.org/10.1111/j.1743-6109.2012.02649.x.
11. Bach LE, Mortimer JA, VandeWeerd C, Corvin J. The association of physical and mental health with sexual activity in older adults in a retirement community. J Sex Med. 2013;10(11):2671–8. https://doi.org/10.1111/jsm.12308.

12. World Health Organization. Defining sexual health: Report of a technical consultation on sexual health. 2006. https://www.who.int/reproductivehealth/topics/gender_rights/defining_sexual_health/en/.
13. Vanwesenbeeck I, ten Have M, de Graaf R. Associations between common mental disorders and sexual dissatisfaction in the general population. Br J Psychiatry. 2014;205(2):151–7. https://doi.org/10.1192/bjp.bp.113.135335.
14. Zemishlany Z, Weizman A. The impact of mental illness on sexual dysfunction. Adv Psychosom Med. 2008;29:89–106. https://doi.org/10.1159/000126626.
15. Christensen BS, Grønbaek M, Osler M, Pedersen BV, Graugaard C, Frisch M. Associations between physical and mental health problems and sexual dysfunctions in sexually active Danes. J Sex Med. 2011;8(7):1890–902. https://doi.org/10.1111/j.1743-6109.2010.02145.x.
16. Palacios-Ceña D, Carrasco-Garrido P, Hernández-Barrera V, Alonso-Blanco C, Jiménez-García R, Fernández-de-las-Peñas C. Sexual behaviors among older adults in Spain: results from a population-based national sexual health survey. J Sex Med. 2012;9(1):121–9. https://doi.org/10.1111/j.1743-6109.2011.02511.x.
17. Lee DM, Nazroo J, O'Connor DB, Blake M, Pendleton N. Sexual health and well-being among older men and women in England: findings from the English longitudinal study of ageing. Arch Sex Behav. 2016a;45(1):133–44. https://doi.org/10.1007/s10508-014-0465-1.
18. Zhang Y, Liu H. A National Longitudinal Study of partnered sex, relationship quality, and mental health among older adults. J Gerontol B Psychol Sci Soc Sci. 2020;75(8):1772–82. https://doi.org/10.1093/geronb/gbz074.
19. Laumann EO, Paik A, Glasser DB, Kang J-H, Wang T, Levinson B, Moreira ED, Nicolosi A, Gingell C. A cross-national study of subjective sexual well-being among older women and men: findings from the global study of sexual attitudes and Behaviors. Arch Sex Behav. 2006;35(2):145–61. https://doi.org/10.1007/s10508-005-9005-3.
20. Dfarhud D, Malmir M, Khanahmadi M. Happiness & health: the biological factors-systematic review article. Iran J Public Health. 2014;43(11):1468–77.
21. Orr J, Layte R, O'Leary N. Sexual activity and relationship quality in middle and older age: findings from the Irish longitudinal study on ageing (TILDA). J Gerontol B Psychol Sci Soc Sci. 2019;74(2):287–97. https://doi.org/10.1093/geronb/gbx038.
22. Hyde Z, Flicker L, Hankey GJ, Almeida OP, McCaul KA, Chubb SAP, Yeap BB. Prevalence of sexual activity and associated factors in men aged 75 to 95 years: a cohort study. Ann Intern Med. 2010;153(11):693–702. https://doi.org/10.7326/0003-4819-153-11-201012070-00002.
23. Lindau ST, Schumm LP, Laumann EO, Levinson W, O'Muircheartaigh CA, Waite LJ. A study of sexuality and health among older adults in the United States. N Engl J Med. 2007;357(8):762–74. https://doi.org/10.1056/NEJMoa067423.
24. Rosen RC, Wing R, Schneider S, Gendrano N. Epidemiology of erectile dysfunction: the role of medical comorbidities and lifestyle factors. Urol Clin North Am. 2005;32(4):403–17, v. https://doi.org/10.1016/j.ucl.2005.08.004.
25. Patten SB. Long-term medical conditions and major depression in the Canadian population. Can J Psychiatry. 1999;44(2):151–7. https://doi.org/10.1177/070674379904400205.
26. Anderson RM. Positive sexuality and its impact on overall well-being. Bundesgesundheitsblatt Gesundheitsforschung Gesundheitsschutz. 2013;56(2):208–14. https://doi.org/10.1007/s00103-012-1607-z.
27. Pick S, Givaudan M, Kline KF. VIII. Sexual pleasure as a key component of integral sexual health. Fem Psychol. 2005;15(1):44–9. https://doi.org/10.1177/0959353505049703.
28. Sprecher S. Sexual satisfaction in premarital relationships: associations with satisfaction, love, commitment, and stability. J Sex Res. 2002;39(3):190–6. https://doi.org/10.1080/00224490209552141.
29. Kleinstäuber M. Factors associated with sexual health and well being in older adulthood. Curr Opin Psychiatry. 2017;30(5):358–68. https://doi.org/10.1097/YCO.0000000000000354.
30. Træen B, Štulhofer A, Janssen E, Carvalheira AA, Hald GM, Lange T, Graham C. Sexual activity and sexual satisfaction among older adults in four European countries. Arch Sex Behav. 2019;48(3):815–29. https://doi.org/10.1007/s10508-018-1256-x.

31. Smith L, Yang L, Veronese N, Soysal P, Stubbs B, Jackson SE. Sexual activity is associated with greater enjoyment of life in older adults. Sex Med. 2019a;7(1):11–8. https://doi.org/10.1016/j.esxm.2018.11.001.
32. DeLamater J, Karraker A. Sexual functioning in older adults. Curr Psychiatry Rep. 2009;11(1):6–11. https://doi.org/10.1007/s11920-009-0002-4.
33. Lee DM, Vanhoutte B, Nazroo J, Pendleton N. Sexual health and positive subjective well-being in partnered older men and women. J Gerontol B Psychol Sci Soc Sci. 2016b;71(4):698–710. https://doi.org/10.1093/geronb/gbw018.
34. Erens B, Mitchell KR, Gibson L, Datta J, Lewis R, Field N, Wellings K. Health status, sexual activity and satisfaction among older people in Britain: a mixed methods study. PLoS One. 2019;14(3):e0213835. https://doi.org/10.1371/journal.pone.0213835.
35. Wellings K, Johnson AM. Framing sexual health research: adopting a broader perspective. Lancet (London, England). 2013;382(9907):1759–62. https://doi.org/10.1016/S0140-6736(13)62378-8.
36. Ridley C, Ogolsky B, Payne P, Totenhagen C, Cate R. Sexual expression: its emotional context in heterosexual, gay, and lesbian couples. J Sex Res. 2008;45(3):305–14. https://doi.org/10.1080/00224490802204449.
37. Gott M, Hinchliff S. How important is sex in later life? The views of older people. Soc Sci Med. 2003;56(8):1617–28. https://doi.org/10.1016/s0277-9536(02)00180-6.
38. Kenny R. A review of the literature on sexual development of older adults in relation to the asexual stereotype of older adults. Can J Fam Youth (Le Journal Canadien De Famille Et De La Jeunesse). 2013;5(1):91–106. https://doi.org/10.29173/cjfy18949.
39. Sharpe TH. Introduction to sexuality in late life. Fam J. 2004;12(2):199–205. https://doi.org/10.1177/0022167804264106.
40. Adams M, Oye J, Parker T. Sexuality of older adults and the internet: from sex education to cybersex. Sex Relat Ther. 2003;18(3):405–15. https://doi.org/10.1080/1468199031000153991.
41. Beckman N, Waern M, Östling S, Sundh V, Skoog I. Determinants of sexual activity in four birth cohorts of Swedish 70-year-olds examined 1971-2001. J Sex Med. 2014;11(2):401–10. https://doi.org/10.1111/jsm.12381.
42. Field N, Mercer CH, Sonnenberg P, Tanton C, Clifton S, Mitchell KR, Erens B, Macdowall W, Wu F, Datta J, Jones KG, Stevens A, Prah P, Copas AJ, Phelps A, Wellings K, Johnson AM. Associations between health and sexual lifestyles in Britain: findings from the third National Survey of sexual attitudes and lifestyles (Natsal-3). Lancet. 2013;382(9907):1830–44. https://doi.org/10.1016/S0140-6736(13)62222-9.
43. DeLamater J, Sill M. Sexual desire in later life. J Sex Res. 2005;42(2):138–49. https://doi.org/10.1080/00224490509552267.
44. Ševčíková A, Sedláková T. The role of sexual activity from the perspective of older adults: a qualitative study. Arch Sex Behav. 2020;49(3):969–81. https://doi.org/10.1007/s10508-019-01617-6.
45. Equality Authority. Implementing equality for lesbians, gays and bisexuals. 2002.
46. Griffin H. Their own received them not: African American lesbians and gays in black churches. Theol Sex. 2000;2000(12):88–100. https://doi.org/10.1177/135583580000601206.
47. Hall WJ, Rodgers GK. Teachers' attitudes toward homosexuality and the lesbian, gay, bisexual, and queer community in the United States. Soc Psychol Educ. 2019;22(1):23–41. https://doi.org/10.1007/s11218-018-9463-9.
48. Grant, J. M. (2011). Injustice at every turn: a report of the national transgender discrimination survey.
49. Safer JD, Coleman E, Feldman J, Garofalo R, Hembree W, Radix A, Sevelius J. Barriers to healthcare for transgender individuals. Curr Opin Endocrinol Diabetes Obes. 2016;23(2):168–71. https://doi.org/10.1097/MED.0000000000000227.
50. Shiu C, Kim H-J, Fredriksen-Goldsen K. Health care engagement among LGBT older adults: the role of depression diagnosis and symptomatology. Gerontologist. 2017;57(suppl 1):S105–14. https://doi.org/10.1093/geront/gnw186.
51. World Health Organization. (2017). World population ageing: highlights report.

52. Choi SK, Meyer IH. LGBT aging: a review of research findings, needs and policy implications. Los Angeles, CA: The Williams Institute; 2016.
53. Jennings L, Barcelos C, McWilliams C, Malecki K. Inequalities in lesbian, gay, bisexual, and transgender (LGBT) health and health care access and utilization in Wisconsin. Prev Med Rep. 2019;14:100864. https://doi.org/10.1016/j.pmedr.2019.100864.
54. Hickson F. Mental health inequalities among gay and bisexual men in England, Scotland and Wales: a large community-based cross-sectional survey. J Public Health. 2016;39(2):266.
55. Marti-Pastor M, Perez G, German D, Pont A, Garin O, Alonso J, Gotsens M, Ferrer M. Health-related quality of life inequalities by sexual orientation: results from the Barcelona health interview survey. PLoS One. 2018;13(1):e0191334. https://doi.org/10.1371/journal.pone.0191334.
56. Dai H, Meyer IH. A population study of health status among sexual minority older adults in select U.S. geographic regions. Health Educ Behav. 2019;46(3):426–35. https://doi.org/10.1177/1090198118818240.
57. Farmer DF, Yancu CN. Hospice and palliative Care for Older Lesbian, gay, bisexual and transgender adults: the effect of history, discrimination, health disparities and legal issues on addressing service needs. Palliat Med Hosp Care Open J. 2015;1(2):36–43. https://doi.org/10.17140/PMHCOJ-1-107.
58. Searle J. Compulsory heterosexuality and lesbian invisibility in nursing. Creat Nurs. 2019;25(2):121–5. https://doi.org/10.1891/1078-4535.25.2.121.
59. Testa RJ, Habarth J, Peta J, Balsam K, Bockting W. Development of the gender minority stress and resilience measure. Psychol Sex Orientat Gend Divers. 2015;2(1):65–77. https://doi.org/10.1037/sgd0000081.
60. Meyer IH. Resilience in the study of minority stress and health of sexual and gender minorities. Psychol Sex Orientat Gend Divers. 2015;2(3):209–13. https://doi.org/10.1037/sgd0000132.
61. de Vries. Aspects of life and death, grief and loss in lesbian, gay, bisexual and transgender communities. 2009.
62. Fredriksen-Goldsen KI, Emlet CA, Kim H-J, Muraco A, Erosheva EA, Goldsen J, Hoy-Ellis CP. The physical and mental health of lesbian, gay male, and bisexual (LGB) older adults: the role of key health indicators and risk and protective factors. Gerontologist. 2013;53(4):664–75. https://doi.org/10.1093/geront/gns123.
63. Diener E, Seligman MEP. Very happy people. Psychol Sci. 2002;13(1):81–4. https://doi.org/10.1111/1467-9280.00415.
64. Wight RG, LeBlanc AJ, de Vries B, Detels R. Stress and mental health among midlife and older gay-identified men. Am J Public Health. 2012;102(3):503–10. https://doi.org/10.2105/AJPH.2011.300384.
65. Fredriksen-Goldsen KI, Kim H-J, Shiu C, Goldsen J, Emlet CA. Successful aging among LGBT older adults: physical and mental health-related quality of life by age group. Gerontologist. 2015;55(1):154–68. https://doi.org/10.1093/geront/gnu081.
66. Grabovac I, Smith L, McDermott DT, Stefanac S, Yang L, Veronese N, Jackson SE. Well-being among older gay and bisexual men and women in England: a cross-sectional population study. J Am Med Dir Assoc. 2019;20(9):1080–1085.e1. https://doi.org/10.1016/j.jamda.2019.01.119.
67. Smith RW, Altman JK, Meeks S, Hinrichs KL. Mental health care for LGBT older adults in long-term care settings: competency, training, and barriers for mental health providers. Clin Gerontol. 2019b;42(2):198–203. https://doi.org/10.1080/07317115.2018.1485197.
68. Reyes ME. Mental health status and attitudes toward aging of lesbian and gay Filipino older adults. N Am J Psychol. 2018;20(1):211.
69. Fredriksen-Goldsen KI, Jen S, Muraco A. Iridescent life course: LGBTQ aging research and blueprint for the future—a systematic review. Gerontology. 2019;65(3):253–74. https://doi.org/10.1159/000493559.
70. Lyons A, Alba B, Waling A, Minichiello V, Hughes M, Barrett C, Fredriksen-Goldsen K, Savage T, Edmonds S. Assessing the combined effect of ageism and sexuality-related stigma on the mental health and well-being of older lesbian and gay adults. Aging Ment Health. 2021:1–10. https://doi.org/10.1080/13607863.2021.1978927.

71. Robinson JG, Molzahn AE. Sexuality and quality of life. J Gerontol Nurs. 2007;33(3):19–27; quiz 38-9. https://doi.org/10.3928/00989134-20070301-05.
72. Mellor RM, Greenfield SM, Dowswell G, Sheppard JP, Quinn T, McManus RJ. Health care professionals' views on discussing sexual wellbeing with patients who have had a stroke: a qualitative study. PLoS One. 2013;8(10):e78802. https://doi.org/10.1371/journal.pone.0078802.
73. Bauer M, Haesler E, Fetherstonhaugh D. Let's talk about sex: older people's views on the recognition of sexuality and sexual health in the health-care setting. Health Expect. 2016;19(6):1237–50. https://doi.org/10.1111/hex.12418.
74. Gledhill S, Schweitzer RD. Sexual desire, erectile dysfunction and the biomedicalization of sex in older heterosexual men. J Adv Nurs. 2014;70(4):894–903. https://doi.org/10.1111/jan.12256.
75. Bauer M, Fetherstonhaugh D, Tarzia L, Nay R, Wellman D, Beattie E. 'I always look under the bed for a man'. Needs and barriers to the expression of sexuality in residential aged care: the views of residents with and without dementia. Psychol Sex. 2013;4(3):296–309. https://doi.org/10.1080/19419899.2012.713869.
76. Lichtenberg PA. Sexuality and physical intimacy in long-term care. Occup Ther Health Care. 2014;28(1):42–50. https://doi.org/10.3109/07380577.2013.865858.
77. Silva R, Candeias A, Santos S, Sá LO, Araújo BR. Mental health, sexuality and old age. J Nurs Socioenviron Health. 2014;1(2):181–9. https://doi.org/10.15696/2358-9884/jonse.v1n2p181-189.
78. Freak-Poli R, Kirkman M, de Castro Lima G, Direk N, Franco OH, Tiemeier H. Sexual activity and physical tenderness in older adults: cross-sectional prevalence and associated characteristics. J Sex Med. 2017;14(7):918–27. https://doi.org/10.1016/j.jsxm.2017.05.010.
79. Fileborn B, Thorpe R, Hawkes G, Minichiello V, Pitts M, Dune T. Sex, desire and pleasure: considering the experiences of older Australian women. Sex Relatsh Ther. 2015;30(1):117–30. https://doi.org/10.1080/14681994.2014.936722.
80. Clayton AH, Alkis AR, Parikh NB, Votta JG. Sexual dysfunction due to psychotropic medications. Psychiatr Clin North Am. 2016;39(3):427–63. https://doi.org/10.1016/j.psc.2016.04.006.
81. Gartlehner G, Thieda P, Hansen RA, Gaynes BN, Deveaugh-Geiss A, Krebs EE, Lohr KN. Comparative risk for harms of second-generation antidepressants: a systematic review and meta-analysis. Drug Saf. 2008;31(10):851–65. https://doi.org/10.2165/00002018-200831100-00004.
82. Serretti A, Chiesa A. A meta-analysis of sexual dysfunction in psychiatric patients taking antipsychotics. Int Clin Psychopharmacol. 2011;26(3):130–40. https://doi.org/10.1097/YIC.0b013e328341e434.
83. Montejo AL, Montejo L, Navarro-Cremades F. Sexual side-effects of antidepressant and antipsychotic drugs. Curr Opin Psychiatry. 2015;28(6):418–23. https://doi.org/10.1097/YCO.0000000000000198.
84. Serretti A, Chiesa A. Treatment-emergent sexual dysfunction related to antidepressants: a meta-analysis. J Clin Psychopharmacol. 2009;29(3):259–66. https://doi.org/10.1097/JCP.0b013e3181a5233f.
85. Wenzel-Seifert K, Ostermaier C-P, Conca A, Haen E. Sexuelle Funktionsstörungen unter antidepressiver Pharmakotherapie. Psychopharmakotherapie. 2015;22:205–11. https://www.ppt-online.de/heftarchiv/2015/04/sexuelle-funktionsstoerungen-unter-antidepressiver-pharmakotherapie.html.
86. Chokka PR, Hankey JR. Assessment and management of sexual dysfunction in the context of depression. Therapeut Adv Psychopharmacol. 2018;8(1):13–23. https://doi.org/10.1177/2045125317720642.
87. Schmidt HM, Hagen M, Kriston L, Soares-Weiser K, Maayan N, Berner MM. Management of sexual dysfunction due to antipsychotic drug therapy. Cochrane Database Syst Rev. 2012;11:CD003546. https://doi.org/10.1002/14651858.CD003546.pub3.
88. Allen K, Baban A, Munjiza J, Pappa S. Management of antipsychotic-related sexual dysfunction: systematic review. J Sex Med. 2019;16(12):1978–87. https://doi.org/10.1016/j.jsxm.2019.08.022.

89. Conaglen HM, Conaglen JV. Drug-induced sexual dysfunction in men and women. Aust Prescr. 2013;36(2):42–5. https://doi.org/10.18773/austprescr.2013.021.
90. Assem-Hilger E, Kasper S. Psychopharmaka und sexuelle Dysfunktion. J Neurol Neurochir Psychiatr. 2005;2(6):30–6. https://www.kup.at/kup/pdf/5258.pdf
91. Knegtering H, van der Moolen A, Castelein S, Kluiter H, van den Bosch RJ. What are the effects of antipsychotics on sexual dysfunctions and endocrine functioning? Psychoneuroendocrinology. 2003;28:109–23. https://doi.org/10.1016/s0306-4530(02)00130-0.
92. Margherita T, Trinchieri M, Perletti G, Magri V, Stamatiou K, Cai T, Montanari E, Trinchieri A. Erectile and ejaculatory dysfunction associated with use of psychotropic drugs: a systematic review. J Sex Med. 2021;18(8):1354–63. https://doi.org/10.1016/j.jsxm.2021.05.016.
93. Montejo AL, Prieto N, de Alarcón R, Casado-Espada N, La Iglesia J, Montejo L. Management strategies for antidepressant-related sexual dysfunction: a clinical approach. J Clin Med. 2019;8(10):1640. https://doi.org/10.3390/jcm8101640.
94. Taylor MJ, Rudkin L, Bullemor-Day P, Lubin J, Chukwujekwu C, Hawton K. Strategies for managing sexual dysfunction induced by antidepressant medication. Cochrane Database Syst Rev. 2013;5:CD003382. https://doi.org/10.1002/14651858.CD003382.pub3.
95. Moura N, Esteves-Sousa D, Halpern C, Farias R, Oliveira-Facucho J, Simião H. HP-2-4 antipsychotic-induced sexual dysfunction revisited. J Sex Med. 2020;17(6):S157–8. https://doi.org/10.1016/j.jsxm.2020.04.118.
96. Rothmore J. Antidepressant-induced sexual dysfunction. Med J Aust. 2020;212(7):329–34. https://doi.org/10.5694/mja2.50522.
97. Lorenz T, Rullo J, Faubion S. Antidepressant-induced female sexual dysfunction. Mayo Clin Proc. 2016;91(9):1280–6. https://doi.org/10.1016/j.mayocp.2016.04.033.

Sexual Activity and Psychosocial Benefits in Older Adults: Challenges and Ways Forward

Siniša Grabovac and Radhika Seiler-Ramadas

5.1 Introduction

Human sexuality is a multidimensional and complex phenomenon that is predominantly influenced by biological, psychological, social, political, cultural, and spiritual factors that constantly interact with one another. The World Health Organization considers sexuality and sexual health as "…*a central aspect of being human, encompassing sex, gender identities and roles, sexual orientation, eroticism, pleasure, intimacy and reproduction…*". Throughout the human lifespan sexuality plays an important role in the lives of individuals, as "…s*exuality is experienced and expressed in thoughts, fantasies, desires, beliefs, attitudes, values, behaviours, practices, roles and relationships…*" [1, 2]. Nevertheless, despite sexuality embracing all of these aspects, not all of them are always felt or conveyed because they may change over time. For instance, desire, reproduction, and attachment are three interrelated but different dimensions of sexuality that vary in importance and intensity as one age [3].

In its *World report on ageing and health,* the World Health Organization defined an older adult as a person who is at least 60 years old [4]. However, this definition differs from low to high income countries. In countries with gross national income per capita the definition of older adults tends to relate to the age upon retirement, which in most wealthier countries is around 65 years [5].

S. Grabovac (✉)
Institute for Outcomes Research—Centre for Medical Statistics, Informatics and Intelligent Systems, Medical University of Vienna, Vienna, Austria
e-mail: sinisa.stefanac@meduniwien.ac.at; sinisa.s.grabovac@gmail.com

R. Seiler-Ramadas
Department of Social and Preventive Medicine, Centre for Public Health, Medical University of Vienna, Vienna, Austria
e-mail: radhika.seiler-ramadas@meduniwien.ac.at

© Springer Nature Switzerland AG 2023
L. Smith, I. Grabovac (eds.), *Sexual Behaviour and Health in Older Adults*, Practical Issues in Geriatrics, https://doi.org/10.1007/978-3-031-21029-7_5

5.2 Sexual Activity Experienced by Older Adults

5.2.1 Perceptions of Sexuality

Whatever the definition of older age may be, sexuality is an important aspect of healthy ageing [6]. There is a growing body of evidence on how older adults define sexual activity and sexual satisfaction. For older adults, the fulfilment of basic emotional and attachment-related needs such as feeling safe, secure, and accepted, as well as becoming more engaged in sexual and intimate contacts turns out to be very important [3]. While healthy and satisfying sexual activity for older people may vary, it is as important for their quality of life as it is for the younger population [7–10]. Sexual activity in older adults is primarily influenced by their own health or illness as well as of their partners, but other aspects such as physical, psychological, and social factors also play a crucial role. Human sexuality is frequently misunderstood in the older population. There is a common worldwide misconception among young-, middle- and many old-aged people that individuals become asexual as they get older [7, 11, 12].

Some empirical studies have even indicated that older adults report less sexual activity, although this may not include cuddling, touching, hugging, and kissing. Sexual expression is however not just limited to sexual intercourse among older adults but can be more varied and diffuse [13]. While for some individuals, sexuality means close companionship, for others it means to touch and be touched. Some older adults associate sexuality with body image, while others associate it with sexual intercourse and activity.

In general, sexual activity can be divided into physical and nonphysical aspects. However, the definition of sexuality in older adults is often broader than that for younger people. Physical aspects include the ability to have penetrative sexual intercourse, while nonphysical aspects consist of positive emotions that are associated with intimacy such as joy, interest, amusement, love, and happiness. Even though sexual intercourse and sexual desire may decrease with age, the nonphysical aspects increase among some individuals [14–16].

5.2.2 Sexual Desire

Research shows that sexual desires persist in old age and there is growing evidence to confirm diverse responses to sexual behaviours among the elderly [17–20]. Sexual thoughts and desires are evident but reported levels of desire are lower than those of younger and middle-aged adults [3]. Yet, while some older adults welcome decreased sexual desire, others are still sexually active (or want to be) and find the physical aspects of sexual activities to be as important, pleasurable, and rewarding as the nonphysical aspects [6, 14, 21–25]. Unfortunately, the sexual well-being and sexual needs of many older adults are still being ignored or met with disdain, even though gender differences that influence sexual satisfaction among older adults appear marginal [20].

5.2.3 Forms of Sexual Behaviour in Older Adults

Types of sexual behaviours differ in older adults. For many of them, penetrative sex may not be possible due to physical and psychological problems such as erectile dysfunction, difficulty in holding a sexual position, a slower response to becoming aroused, or increased anxiety that the sexual activity may for instance trigger another heart attack, depression, or sadness [7, 16]. However, those who are able and willing to participate in sexual behaviours and those who are interested in acquiring active sexual pleasure have other options such as touching, hugging, cuddling, kissing, or even mutual genital stroking and/or masturbation [26–28]. The majority of older adults still rely on physical tenderness through which the human touch plays an important role in communication, relationships, and the sharing of feelings between partners. Human touch is considered to be important for maintaining or instigating interpersonal and intimate relationships. The lack of human touch leads to feelings of isolation, anxiety, insecurity, and decreased sensory awareness, all of which can negatively impact human health [5, 29–31].

5.3 Psychosocial Benefits of Sexual Activity in Older Age

Older people, especially those in their transition to retirement, are experiencing a time in which significant changes in their social, physical, and mental health are happening. It is during this time that they feel an acute need for a sense of belonging [32]. The recent Covid-19 pandemic has emphasized social distancing and heightened feelings of loneliness and fear among the older adults that became the most vulnerable part of our population, but also forcing them even further into isolation. It is especially during this time that older people need to feel and stay mentally and physically healthy.

For many elderly people, the ability to have and maintain a sex life as well as having a fulfilling and rewarding sexual experience is perceived to be important to their mental and physical health. Several studies have shown that older adults who had sexual desires were more physically active, reported the lowest number of medical conditions, and took few or no medications [33–36]. This is extremely significant, as it is around this period in life where people are faced with increasing health problems and challenges. It is important to emphasize and advocate the well-being of older people not just to prevent strain on our current healthcare system, but also to espouse comprehensive health among older individuals.

According to the World Health Organization (WHO), health is not merely an absence of disease or infirmity, but "*a state of complete physical, mental and social well-being*" [37]. While still being a relatively unexplored area of research, an increasing number of reviews and studies have nevertheless confirmed that sexual activity and expressions of intimate behaviour are associated with well-being, and that positive sexual activity is linked to a greater enjoyment of life, a higher quality of life in the social domain, higher levels of emotional and physical satisfaction, and greater health and life quality across the lifespan [35, 38–41]. Our psychological, public health, and biomedical efforts to date are clearly focused on reducing risks of factors that are harmful to health and emphasizing prevention and treatment programmes, while health promoting psychosocial assets are under-navigated [42]. Yet, there are modifiable dimensions of psychological well-being uniquely associated with a reduced risk of chronic conditions, a crucial one being positive sexual behaviour [40, 42].

Positive sexual behaviours such as frequent emotional connections and/or enjoyment of sexual intercourse, the ability to communicate well about the sexual aspect of a relationship, as well as enhancing romance and intimacy promote subjective well-being [40, 41]. Touching or holding hands, hugging and kissing, mutual stroking and masturbation, as well as frequent sexual intercourse (bi-monthly or more) are modifiable factors that have been associated with low levels of stress, better health, and positive psychology [38–40]. Likewise, active sex life in older adults has been associated with higher levels of relaxation and reduced depression, increased self-esteem, feelings of being *"normal, strong and alive"* and also with higher relationship satisfaction. It has also been associated with decreased pain sensitivity, better cardiovascular health, lower incidences of chronic airway diseases, better recovery, better management of chronic diseases in general, and lower mortality [11, 38, 43–53]. Overall, a higher frequency of sexual activity is undeniably linked to better mental and physical health. Through greater enjoyment of life and higher levels of emotional and physical satisfaction, essential components of life quality and subjective well-being are realized.

5.4 Challenges Affecting Sexuality in Older Adults

5.4.1 Reasons for Sexual Inactivity

Increased life expectancy can lead to an increased number of health issues and chronic diseases in older adults, which inevitably affect their overall health as well as their sexuality [4, 54]. As human beings age, their bodies and biological functions change. Their psychological, social, physical, and cultural aspects also shift, often negatively affecting their own perceptions of sexuality [55]. Sexual desire may be further impaired by hormonal changes and disease-specific medication [3]. For some older people, these significant life changes create a serious impact on their sexuality, satisfaction, and overall well-being [7].

However, the biggest barrier to being sexually inactive is not older age, but the lack of partner availability, and the presence of one or more health-related long-term and debilitating conditions. These conditions include arthritis, diabetes, fatigue, cancer, cardiovascular, neurological, and psychiatric problems, but may also involve the side effects of medications, relationship issues (e.g. lack of commitment or interest), one's living environment (e.g. institutionalization, lack of privacy), and cultural differences (e.g. personal attitudes and beliefs towards engagement in sexual activities) [5, 6, 11, 12, 55–59]. Many couples experience changes in their marital status during the course of their lives, resulting in individuals who are not married, those who do not cohabit with their partner anymore, or those who are widowed [60, 61]. Older women are often faced with widowhood, and thus cannot have their emotional needs satisfied. Further physical, biological, and age-related changes make it conceivable that older adults engage in less sexual activity with age [3]. Other psychological factors such as concerns about body image, embarrassment, fear, loneliness, diminished self-esteem, and self-consciousness regarding the ability to sexually satisfy their partners are also likely to affect interpersonal communication and negatively influence sexual behaviours and sexual satisfaction [26, 62–68]. Effectively addressing sexual behaviours among older adults and understanding their need to be sexually active can contribute to maintaining and improving their well-being and quality of life [5, 60, 69].

Some older adults will have minor health issues or none at all, while others will require full-time assistance on an everyday basis for their basic needs. Reduced sexual desire, behaviour, and participation in sexual activities are known to decrease with rapidly deteriorating health and can differ markedly among the elderly [51, 70, 71]. Clearly, the health of one's partner is important, and when considering health status among older adults, having a physically and mentally healthy partner goes hand in hand with more sexual activity [3].

5.4.2 Social and Cultural Contexts

Education, physical health, and psychosocial well-being are important personal resources that determine how people experience the various aspects of sexuality into and across old age [3]. However, attitudes, traditions, patterns, norms, and beliefs towards sexuality in later life especially with regard to older adults vary across different ethnic, religious, and cultural backgrounds. For instance, cultural stereotypes that older people are asexual or sexually inactive individuals may in fact make them feel more apprehensive about sexual activity [13]. Among older women, traditional views of sexuality such as beliefs that women are subordinate and should wait for the man to initiate sexual activity or that sex is linked to reproduction, marriage, or prostitution may be factors that discourage them from sexual re-engagement [13].

There is very limited evidence and knowledge about the relationship between sexual satisfaction and religiosity in older adults [72]. However, some findings confirm that older men and women who are religious are typically more sexually conservative regardless of their educational level [73]. Religious teachings often place a strong emphasis on the procreative function of sex and seem to continuously discourage the dissemination of accurate sexual knowledge within families as well as educational structures, thereby leading to de-sexualization, misinformation, prejudice, and stigmatization of sexual activity in older age. In societies where religious belief about sexual activity is based on procreation (e.g. the Catholic church), widows or widowers often view their sex life as being over and do not want to find a new intimate partner or husband.

Hence for many older adults, the individual, structural, and social contexts in which they grew up may have negatively shaped their current beliefs about sexual behaviours. Sex may never have been discussed openly, sexual activity was thought to be reserved only for the young, sex for pleasure was perceived as unacceptable, and masturbation for both men and women was considered taboo and shameful in their culture [23, 74, 75]. These beliefs and perceptions still exist in many cultures.

Cultural factors play a significant role in people's lives and it is very difficult to separate these from the individual or their social context. Culture and race can also influence help-seeking behaviour related to sexual health [76]. Thus, in order to understand sexual expression, sexual desires, behaviours, and sexual activities in older adults, an interdisciplinary and open discussion on sexuality together with cultural, ethnic, and religious sensitivity is needed [5].

5.4.3 Structural Challenges

Identity roles, lifestyle characteristics, and factors such as where one grew up affect one's perceptions of sexuality as much as structural factors such as the lack of privacy [11, 23, 44, 77, 78]. For instance, the lack of privacy in nursing homes or assisted living facilities can be a major obstacle to sexual expression. Nursing homes and assisted living facilities are two types of senior centres that are different in the nature of care for their residents. The difference being that in nursing homes constant monitoring and a round-the-clock medical care are frequently required as their residents often have severe healthcare conditions. On the other hand, in assisted living facilities (also called retirement homes) only basic supervision or minimal to moderate care such as housekeeping, laundry, mobile transfers, or some guidance for their residents is all that is needed. In such facilities round-the-clock medical monitoring and medical staff are not always available.

Despite these differences, there still exists a lack of privacy in both structures, as rooms are usually always shared with sometimes two or more other occupants. Unsurprisingly, under these circumstances performing sexual activities or having intimate time with another person rarely happens [13]. Moreover, the structure of these facilities is primarily organized around healthcare provision (such as bathing, dressing, or the administration of medication), mealtimes, and numerous social and physical activities which discourage residents from staying in their rooms. Some studies have also reported that varying degrees of control from staff members such as regular and sudden room checks, no lock policies, and restrictive behaviours exist in such facilities, which significantly hinder their residents' perceptions of privacy and naturally discourage or prevent them from sexual expression or sexual activity [79–83].

Nonetheless, sexual behaviours do exist in nursing homes, the most common being handholding, hugging, kissing, and masturbation [84]. Despite common knowledge that sexual activity is a private act between consenting adults, the impact of institutional monitoring, rules, and policies as well as the attitude of staff towards residents on their sexuality is often negative [82, 85–90]. Such environments present barriers to the sexual expression and sexual acts of residents. Hence, when promoting sexual culture comfortably and safely, these facts must be taken into consideration. Findings such as these should initiate discussions in private homes, in nursing and assisted living facilities, as well as in other institutions that lead to strategies in facilitating better sexual health and recognizing sexual needs among older adults.

The United Nations' principles for older persons clearly state that privacy is a fundamental right for all human beings regardless of their health and social background [91]. Thus, privacy needs must be acknowledged and offered to residents in the most appropriate and effective way [88]. Additionally, it is important to create a comfortable, safe, and supportive environment that permits sexual expression, promotes sexual culture, and comfortably deals with concerns on sexuality. It is vital to adopt new policies or modify existing ones and educate family members as well as healthcare providers in using a holistic approach to the sexual rights, benefits, and possibilities for their elderly family member or resident. It is important to note that discriminatory or patronizing attitudes from family or staff members are often influenced by their own levels of comfort as well as organizational policies where sexual expression and acts are seen as inappropriate. Frailty, illness, cultural and religious assumptions, the lack of education, and sexually related false information are further reasons for hostile attitudes. A facility that is not tolerant towards the sexual needs of elderly or has strict rules to residents' sexual needs will inevitably have a negative impact on the attitudes and behaviour of their staff. Studies have shown that a lack of sexual expression and interpersonal intimacy can lead to social isolation, a lack of fulfilment in life, loneliness, and reduced self-esteem, but it can also subjectively constrain mental health. Nevertheless, few studies have stressed that educating family and staff members about sexual well-being in older adults can elicit supportive environments, generate positive attitudes, and effectively address their sexuality [92, 93]. Educating staff and family members should not only focus on the area of sexuality but should also acknowledge and understand basic human needs with regard to values, beliefs, traditions, culture, and religion. Figure 5.1 addresses some of the ideas and practical recommendations that are necessary for promoting sexual well-being in older adults.

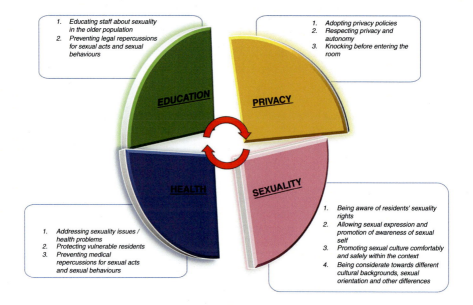

Fig. 5.1 Holistic approach towards sexuality in residence facilities

5.5 Strategies to Help Support Sexuality in Older Adults

5.5.1 Healthcare Practitioners

From the healthcare perspective, relationships between normative sexual values, practices, and beliefs that could prevent or enhance sexual life should be examined within specific contexts and circumstances in order to better understand the sexual behaviour of older people [94]. For instance, practitioners should be aware that there could be a mismatch between the desire for sex and physical barriers to enjoying sex among some of their patients and plan appropriate interventions. To describe the importance of this, in one study 13% of women between 67 and 71 years of age were reported to avoid sexual activity due to sexual problems. Although this group of women had the lowest lack of interest in sex rates, they had the highest rates of vaginal dryness and pain with intercourse [76].

Through understanding the social reality among older people, unmet needs in sexual healthcare services for later life can be better addressed. Prevailing evidence shows that assumptions of asexuality among older adults and clinicians' lack of knowledge of sexual health issues for this age group add to communication gaps around sexual health between clinicians and older adults [95]. This is noteworthy, as healthcare professionals are known to avoid discussing sex with older adults. It is important for healthcare providers to provide more consideration to the sexual needs of older adults by recognizing the importance of sexual activity and its direct relationship to life quality [96]. As sexual health was reported as a highly important aspect of life quality among people with both poor and good health, sexual health should be a routine part of clinicians' assessments of their patients [97]. Due to personal, cultural, or religious beliefs, older adults do not always seek help for sexual difficulties [98–100].

All healthcare professionals and staff who are taking care of older adults should encourage older individuals to seek help should they need it. It is important to properly acknowledge and address the sexual needs of older adults through open and safe discussions. This can be done by active listening and providing holistic and multidisciplinary professional advice and medical help. It can further be improved through developing sexual health programmes that encourage a lifestyle of empowerment, as studies have shown that such positive behaviours can contribute to the maintenance and improvement of individuals' overall quality of life and their wellbeing [5, 17, 54, 60, 69, 101].

5.5.2 Sexuality Education, Sexually Transmitted Infections, and Condom Use

People with higher education may have more positive attitudes towards sexuality in the later stages of their lives. Although this evidence is not conclusive, more educated people have reported slightly more sexual activity, sexual thoughts, and sexual intimacy [3]. Furthermore, sexuality education interventions have been shown to increase knowledge, satisfaction, and sexual activity among older adults, while dispelling negative myths, stereotypes, and self-fulfilling attitudes [13].

Older adults generally dislike condom use but are just as vulnerable to contracting sexually transmitted infections (STIs) [94]. In fact, the rates of STIs have been increasing among older individuals globally for the last 20 years, hence underscoring the importance of safer sex awareness and practices among them [95, 96]. Evidently, there is a gap in knowledge of STIs among older adults as well as that of the social contexts in which this knowledge is acquired [94, 95]. Many older adults have experienced limited information about sex as they were growing up or may have faced moral undertones and a lack of clarity about sexuality and sexual experiences from their caregivers. Older people grew up at a time when comprehensive sexuality education was unavailable in schools, and sex was a taboo theme, while STIs were stigmatized [96]. Hence, there exists gendered stigma and marginalization of risk groups among many older adults, as well as the perception that sexual activity is safe from STIs in long-term relationships [95].

There is the perception that using condoms reduces sexual pleasure, and is irrelevant to older adults, since condoms are generally targeted to people of reproductive age [94]. Cultural and generational differences where women are used to male-dominant sexual scripts may also make condom negotiation skills difficult and uncomfortable for women [96]. However, where risky sexual practices still continue in later life, or where re-partnering occurs after the death or divorce of a spouse, the use of condoms is ever more relevant to sexually active older adults [94, 96].

5.6 Conclusion and Future Prospects

Although sexuality is very diverse, it represents an important aspect of active ageing. Sexual needs and behaviours are influenced by a constant interaction of individual characteristics that are influenced by lifestyle, education, biology, and psychology, as well as social, political, cultural, and spiritual aspects. The fulfilment of basic emotional and attachment-related needs in older adults is as important as it is for the younger population. While not every older adult will wish to have sexual intercourse, there are many to whom being intimate is equally important for a healthy and inspiring life.

While communication, relationships, and the sharing of feelings between partners play an important role for one's well-being and quality of life, other types of sexual behaviours might be just as important. Physical tenderness, handholding, hugging, cuddling, kissing, mutual genital stroking, masturbation as well as penetrative sex are some types of sexual behaviours in older adults that are perceived to be important for mental and physical health.

Unfortunately, many older adults are seen as asexual, and thus their sexual well-being and sexual needs are still being ignored or met with disdain. The biggest barrier is not the old age, but rather a number of other factors such as health problems, relationship issues, the lack of privacy in a living environment, as well as cultural, political, and social differences.

Acknowledging and addressing sexual behaviour among older adults and accepting their need to be sexually active can contribute to maintaining and improving their well-being and quality of life. It is important to create a comfortable, safe, and supportive environment that permits sexual expression, promotes sexual culture, and comfortably deals with sexuality issues. It is also vital to adopt new policies or modify the existing ones as well as to educate family members, healthcare and other service providers about a holistic approach for the elderly and their sexual rights, benefits, and possibilities.

References

1. World Association for Sexual Health. Declaration of sexual rights. 2014. https://worldsexualhealth.net/resources/declaration-of-sexual-rights/. Accessed 31 Aug 2020.
2. World Health Organization. Sexual and reproductive health—defining sexual health. 2006. https://www.who.int/reproductivehealth/topics/sexual_health/sh_definitions/en/. Accessed 31 Aug 2020.
3. Kolodziejczak K, et al. Sexual activity, sexual thoughts, and intimacy among older adults: links with physical health and psychosocial resources for successful aging. Psychol Aging. 2019;34(3):389.
4. World Health Organization. World report on ageing and health. 2015. https://www.who.int/ageing/events/world-report-2015-launch/en/. Accessed 31 Aug 2020.
5. Freak-Poli R. It's not age that prevents sexual activity later in life. Aust J Ageing. 2020;39(Suppl 1):22–9.
6. Graf AS, Patrick JH. The influence of sexual attitudes on mid- to late-life sexual well-being: age, not gender, as a salient factor. Int J Aging Hum Dev. 2014;79(1):55–79.

7. Hinchliff S, et al. Older adults' experiences of sexual difficulties: qualitative findings from the English longitudinal study on ageing (ELSA). J Sex Res. 2018;55(2):152–63.
8. Verschuren JE, et al. Chronic disease and sexuality: a generic conceptual framework. J Sex Res. 2010;47(2):153–70.
9. McNicoll L. Issues of sexuality in the elderly. Med Health R I. 2008;91(10):321–2.
10. Papaharitou S, et al. Factors associated with sexuality in later life: an exploratory study in a group of Greek married older adults. Arch Gerontol Geriatr. 2008;46(2):191–201.
11. DeLamater J. Sexual expression in later life: a review and synthesis. J Sex Res. 2012;49(2–3):125–41.
12. Freak-Poli R, et al. Sexual activity and physical tenderness in older adults: cross-sectional prevalence and associated characteristics. J Sex Med. 2017;14(7):918–27.
13. Deacon S, Minichiello V, Plummer D. Sexuality and older people: revisiting the assumptions. Educ Gerontol. 1995;21(5):497–513.
14. Waite LJ, et al. Sexuality: measures of partnerships, practices, attitudes, and problems in the National Social Life, health, and Aging study. J Gerontol B Psychol Sci Soc Sci. 2009;64(Suppl 1):i56–66.
15. Hinchliff S, Gott M. Perceptions of well-being in sexual ill health: what role does age play? J Health Psychol. 2004;9(5):649–60.
16. Bouman WP. The Oxford textbook of old age psychiatry. In: Dening T, Thomas A, editors. Sexuality in later life. Oxford: Oxford University Press; 2013. p. 703–23.
17. Heidari S. Sexuality and older people: a neglected issue. Reprod Health Matters. 2016;24(48):1–5.
18. Lindau ST, et al. A study of sexuality and health among older adults in the United States. N Engl J Med. 2007;357(8):762–74.
19. Beckman N, et al. Secular trends in self reported sexual activity and satisfaction in Swedish 70 year olds: cross sectional survey of four populations, 1971-2001. BMJ. 2008;337:a279.
20. Træen B, et al. Sexuality in older adults (65+)—an overview of the recent literature, part 2: body Image and sexual satisfaction. Int J Sex Health. 2017;29(1):11–21.
21. Muller B, et al. Sexuality and affection among elderly German men and women in long-term relationships: results of a prospective population-based study. PLoS One. 2014;9(11):e111404.
22. Ferris JA, et al. Self reported sexual activity in Australian sexagenarians. BMJ. 2008;337:a1250.
23. Fileborn B, et al. Sex, desire and pleasure: considering the experiences of older Australian women. Sex Relat Ther. 2015;30(1):117–30.
24. Lee DM, et al. Sexual health and well-being among older men and women in England: findings from the English longitudinal study of ageing. Arch Sex Behav. 2016;45(1):133–44.
25. Lee DM, et al. Sexual health and positive subjective well-being in partnered older men and Women. J Gerontol B Psychol Sci Soc Sci. 2016;71(4):698–710.
26. Sandberg L. In lust we trust? Masculinity and sexual desire in later life. Men Masculinities. 2016;19(2):192–208.
27. Schlesinger B. The sexless years or sex rediscovered. In: Neugebauer-Visano R, editor. Seniors and sexuality: experiencing intimacy in later life. Toronto: Canadian Scholars' Press; 1995. p. 5–16.
28. Ussher JM, et al. Renegotiating sex and intimacy after cancer: resisting the coital imperative. Cancer Nurs. 2013;36(6):454–62.
29. Bush E. The use of human touch to improve the Well-being of older adults. A holistic nursing intervention. J Holist Nurs. 2001;19(3):256–70.
30. Vieira AI, et al. Hand tactile discrimination, social touch and frailty criteria in elderly people: a cross sectional observational study. Arch Gerontol Geriatr. 2016;66:73–81.
31. Umberson D, Montez JK. Social relationships and health: a flashpoint for health policy. J Health Soc Behav. 2010;51(Suppl):S54–66.
32. Flett GL, Heisel MJ. Aging and feeling valued versus expendable during the COVID-19 pandemic and beyond: a review and commentary of why mattering is fundamental to the health and well-being of older adults. Int J Ment Heal Addict. 2021;19:2443–69.

33. Johnson BK. A correlational framework for understanding sexuality in women age 50 and older. Health Care Women Int. 1998;19(6):553–64.
34. Amin SH, Kuhle CL, Fitzpatrick LA. Comprehensive evaluation of the older woman. Mayo Clin Proc. 2003;78(9):1157–85.
35. Lagana L, Maciel M. Sexual desire among Mexican-American older women: a qualitative study. Cult Health Sex. 2010;12(6):705–19.
36. Seguin RA, et al. Strength training improves body image and physical activity behaviors among midlife and older rural women. J Ext. 2013;51(4):4FEA2.
37. World Health Organization. Constitution of the World Health Organization. 2006. https://www.who.int/about/who-we-are/constitution. Accessed 17 Sep 2020.
38. Syme ML. The evolving concept of older adult sexual behavior and its benefits. Generations. 2014;38:35–41.
39. Flynn T-J, Gow AJ. Examining associations between sexual behaviours and quality of life in older adults. Age Ageing. 2015;44(5):823–8.
40. Smith L, et al. Sexual activity is associated with greater enjoyment of life in older adults. Sex Med. 2019;7(1):11–8.
41. Blumenstock SM, et al. High emotional and sexual satisfaction among partnered Midlife Canadians: associations with relationship characteristics, sexual activity and communication, and health. Arch Sex Behav. 2020;49(3):953–67.
42. Kim ES, Ong A. Characterizing the pathways underlying the association between psychological well-being and health. Innov Aging. 2019;3(Supplement_1):S813.
43. Lindau ST, Gavrilova N. Sex, health, and years of sexually active life gained due to good health: evidence from two US population based cross sectional surveys of ageing. BMJ. 2010;340:c810.
44. Kontula O, Haavio-Mannila E. The impact of aging on human sexual activity and sexual desire. J Sex Res. 2009;46(1):46–56.
45. Brody S. The relative health benefits of different sexual activities. J Sex Med. 2010;7(4 Pt 1):1336–61.
46. Heiman JR, et al. Sexual satisfaction and relationship happiness in midlife and older couples in five countries. Arch Sex Behav. 2011;40(4):741–53.
47. Jannini EA, et al. Is sex just fun? How sexual activity improves health. J Sex Med. 2009;6(10):2640–8.
48. Merghati Khoei E, et al. Development, validity and reliability of sexual health measures for spinal cord injured patients in Iran. Int J Fertil Steril. 2013;7(2):82–7.
49. Nusbaum MR, Hamilton C, Lenahan P. Chronic illness and sexual functioning. Am Fam Physician. 2003;67(2):347–54.
50. Ziaei T, et al. Psychometric properties of the Farsi version of modified multidimensional sexual self-concept questionnaire. Iran J Nurs Midwifery Res. 2013;18(6):439–45.
51. DeLamater JD, Sill M. Sexual desire in later life. J Sex Res. 2005;42(2):138–49.
52. Byers ES. Relationship satisfaction and sexual satisfaction: a longitudinal study of individuals in long-term relationships. J Sex Res. 2005;42(2):113–8.
53. Rosen RC, et al. Men with sexual problems and their partners: findings from the international survey of relationships. Arch Sex Behav. 2016;45(1):159–73.
54. Merghati-Khoei E, et al. Sexuality and elderly with chronic diseases: a review of the existing literature. J Res Med Sci. 2016;21:136.
55. DeLamater J, Karraker A. Sexual functioning in older adults. Curr Psychiatry Rep. 2009;11(1):6–11.
56. Noroozi M, et al. How does a group of Iranian youth conceptualize their risky sexual experiences? Iran Red Crescent Med J. 2015;17(2):e18301.
57. Beckman N, et al. Determinants of sexual activity in four birth cohorts of Swedish 70-year-olds examined 1971–2001. J Sex Med. 2014;11(2):401–10.
58. Jeong HC, et al. Sexual behavior of the elderly in urban areas. World J Mens Health. 2012;30(3):166–71.

59. Træen B, et al. Sexuality in older adults (65+)—an overview of the literature, part 1: sexual function and its difficulties. Int J Sex Health. 2017;29(1):1–10.
60. Karraker A, Delamater J, Schwartz CR. Sexual frequency decline from midlife to later life. J Gerontol B Psychol Sci Soc Sci. 2011;66(4):502–12.
61. George LK, Weiler SJ. Sexuality in middle and late life. The effects of age, cohort, and gender. Arch Gen Psychiatry. 1981;38(8):919–23.
62. Jowett A, Peel E, Shaw RL. Sex and diabetes: a thematic analysis of gay and bisexual men's accounts. J Health Psychol. 2012;17(3):409–18.
63. Potts A, et al. "Viagra stories": challenging 'erectile dysfunction'. Soc Sci Med. 2004;59(3):489–99.
64. Lev EL. Quality of life of men treated with brachytherapies for prostate cancer. Health Qual Life Outcomes. 2004;2:28.
65. Pirl WF, Mello J. Psychological complications of prostate cancer. Oncology (Williston Park). 2002;16(11):1448–53; discussion 1453–4, 1457–8, 1467.
66. Visser A, et al. Changes in health-related quality of life of men with prostate cancer 3 months after diagnosis: the role of psychosocial factors and comparisment with benign prostate hyperplasia patients. Patient Educ Couns. 2003;49(3):225–32.
67. Bokhour BG, et al. Sexuality after treatment for early prostate cancer: exploring the meanings of "erectile dysfunction". J Gen Intern Med. 2001;16(10):649–55.
68. Butler L, et al. Quality of life post radical prostatectomy: a male perspective. Urol Nurs. 2001;21(4):283–8.
69. Rosen RC, Bachmann GA. Sexual well-being, happiness, and satisfaction, in women: the case for a new conceptual paradigm. J Sex Marital Ther. 2008;34(4):291–7; discussion 298-307.
70. Mercer CH, et al. Changes in sexual attitudes and lifestyles in Britain through the life course and over time: findings from the National Surveys of sexual attitudes and lifestyles (Natsal). Lancet. 2013;382(9907):1781–94.
71. Freak-Poli R, et al. Happiness, rather than depression, is associated with sexual behaviour in partnered older adults. Age Ageing. 2017;46(1):101–7.
72. McFarland MJ, Uecker JE, Regnerus MD. The role of religion in shaping sexual frequency and satisfaction: evidence from married and unmarried older adults. J Sex Res. 2011;48(2–3):297–308.
73. Le Gall A, Mullet E, Riviere Shafighi S. Age, religious beliefs, and sexual attitudes. J Sex Res. 2002;39(3):207–16.
74. Lobsenz N. Sex and the senior citizen. New York: Bruner/Mazel; 1974.
75. Butler R, Lewis M. Aging and mental health, vol. 3. Saint Louis, MO: Mosby; 1988.
76. Hughes AK, Rostant OS, Pelon S. Sexual problems among older women by age and race. J Womens Health. 2015;24(8):663–9.
77. Lodge AC, Umberson D. All shook up: sexuality of mid- to later life married couples. J Marriage Fam. 2012;74(3):428–43.
78. Montemurro B, Gillen MM. Wrinkles and sagging flesh: exploring transformations in women's sexual body image. J Women Aging. 2013;25(1):3–23.
79. Calkins M, Cassella C. Exploring the cost and value of private versus shared bedrooms in nursing homes. Gerontologist. 2007;47(2):169–83.
80. Morgan LA. Balancing safety and privacy: the case of room locks in assisted living. J Hous Elder. 2009;23(3):185–203.
81. Bauer M. Their only privacy is between their sheets. Privacy and the sexuality of elderly nursing home residents. J Gerontol Nurs. 1999;25(8):37–41.
82. Rheaume C, Mitty E. Sexuality and intimacy in older adults. Geriatr Nurs. 2008;29(5):342–9.
83. McCartney JR, et al. Sexuality and the institutionalized elderly. J Am Geriatr Soc. 1987;35(4):331–3.
84. Steinke EE. Sexuality in aging: implications for nursing facility staff. J Contin Educ Nurs. 1997;28(2):59–63.
85. Frankowski AC, Clark LJ. Sexuality and intimacy in assisted living: residents' perspectives and experiences. Sex Res Social Policy. 2009;6(4):25–37.

86. Eddy DM. Before and after attitudes toward aging in a BSN program. J Gerontol Nurs. 1986;12(5):30–4.
87. Luketich GF. Sex and the elderly: what do nurses know? Educ Gerontol. 1991;17(6):573–80.
88. Roach SM. Sexual behaviour of nursing home residents: staff perceptions and responses. J Adv Nurs. 2004;48(4):371–9.
89. Hajjar RR, Kamel HK. Sexuality in the nursing home, part 1: attitudes and barriers to sexual expression. J Am Med Dir Assoc. 2004;5(2 Suppl):S42–7.
90. National Resource Center on LGBT Aging. Outing age 2010: public policy issues affecting lesbian, gay, bisexual and transgender elders. 2010. https://www.lgbtagingcenter.org/resources/resource.cfm?r=30. Accessed 15 Sep 2020.
91. Office of the High Commissioner for Human Rights. United Nations principles for older persons. 2020. https://www.ohchr.org/en/professionalinterest/pages/olderpersons.aspx. Accessed 17 Sep 2020.
92. Quinn-Krach P, Van Hoozer H. Sexuality of the aged and the attitudes and knowledge of nursing students. J Nurs Educ. 1988;27(8):359–63.
93. Walker BL, Harrington D. Effects of staff training on staff knowledge and attitudes about sexuality. Educ Gerontol. 2002;28(8):639–54.
94. Agunbiade OM, Togunde D. 'No sweet in sex': perceptions of condom usefulness among elderly Yoruba people in Ibadan Nigeria. J Cross Cult Gerontol. 2018;33(3):319–36.
95. Dalrymple J, et al. Socio-cultural influences upon knowledge of sexually transmitted infections: a qualitative study with heterosexual middle-aged adults in Scotland. Reprod Health Matters. 2016;24(48):34–42.
96. Fileborn B, et al. Safer sex in later life: qualitative interviews with older Australians on their understandings and practices of safer sex. J Sex Res. 2018;55(2):164–77.
97. Flynn KE, et al. Sexual satisfaction and the importance of sexual health to quality of life throughout the life course of US adults. J Sex Med. 2016;13(11):1642–50.
98. Hinchliff S, Gott M. Seeking medical help for sexual concerns in mid- and later life: a review of the literature. J Sex Res. 2011;48(2–3):106–17.
99. Gleser H. Sex, women and the menopause: are specialist trainee doctors up for it? A survey of views and attitudes of specialist trainee doctors in Community Sexual & Reproductive Health and Obstetrics & Gynaecology around sexuality and sexual healthcare in the (peri) menopause. Post Reprod Health. 2015;21(1):26–33.
100. Mellor RM, et al. Health care professionals' views on discussing sexual wellbeing with patients who have had a stroke: a qualitative study. PLoS One. 2013;8(10):e78802.
101. World Health Organization. Sexual health, human rights and the law. 2015. https://www.who.int/reproductivehealth/publications/sexual_health/sexual-health-human-rights-law/en/. Accessed 1 Sep 2020.

'We're Still Here, We're Still Queer, We're Still Doing It': Sex and Sexual Health in Older LGBTQ+ Adults

6

Joshua W. Katz, Lee Smith, and Daragh T. McDermott

While a majority of older adults still identify as heterosexual or straight, in contemporary western society an increasing number of older adults identify as Lesbian, Gay, Bisexual, Transgender, Queer, or Questioning (LGBTQ+; [1–3]). For example, according to Fleishman et al. [4] there are currently three million individuals over the age of 65 who self-identify as LGBTQ residing in the United States—a number, which is higher than the estimated one and a half million in 2010 [5] and is expected to grow to more than five million by 2060. Further, there is the additional possibility of there being another 15 million American adults over the age of 50 who do not explicitly identify as LGBT but who also engage in same-sex sexual behaviours and/or same-sex romantic relationships by that point [6]. Findings from other countries paint a similar picture; for example, as of 2016, there were more than 60,000 adults over the age of 65 who identified as non-heterosexual living in Australia (i.e., 1 to 2% of the Australian adult population aged 65 or more; [7]). Despite such findings, the exact proportion of older sexual and gender minority (SGM) adults is not definitively known in most countries, however.[1] Indeed, reports on the number of older LGBTQ+ adults are based largely on estimates and inferences [9]. Canadian data, for instance, places the number of LGB adults aged 65 or

---

[1] LGBTQ+ people are generally grouped into one of two categories: sexual minority is a general umbrella term that is used to describe persons who do not identify as heterosexual (e.g., gay, lesbian, bisexual) and gender minority, simply stated, is used as a term for someone who does not identify as cisgender (e.g., transgender, nonbinary, gender nonconforming; [8]).

J. W. Katz
Department of Psychology, University of Saskatchewan, Saskatoon, SK, Canada

L. Smith
Center for Health Performance and Wellbeing, Anglia Ruskin University, Cambridge, UK

D. T. McDermott (✉)
NTU Psychology, School of Social Sciences, Nottingham Trent University, Nottingham, UK
e-mail: daragh.mcdermott@ntu.ac.uk

older at anywhere between 98,000 and 396,000 individuals [10]. Not only is this a very broad range based on arguably old data (i.e., the 2011 Canadian census), but the results of this study are also based on extrapolations made from a combination of Canadian and American data, which assumes that the two countries are equivalent. Furthermore, this reliance on American data as a proxy for Canadian numbers highlights how accurate data on the proportion of older LGBTQ+ adults is not available in most (western) countries. Moreover, such estimates are incomplete in that they do not take into account gender minority persons—a common issue in much extant research. While there are any number of potential reasons why estimates and inferences are used to determine the exact number of older LGBTQ+ adults, in large part, the reliance on such methods is the result of SGMs' lifelong experiences of discrimination and prejudice, which have, in turn, resulted in a hesitancy, in particular among older SGM adults, to 'come out of the closet'.

Although attitudes towards LGBTQ+ persons have generally improved over time [11] and legislation has been put in place in certain countries (e.g., the United States) to protect members of the LGBTQ+ community [12], historically, SGM persons have been persecuted on account of their sexual orientation and/or gender identity. For an example of this that is relevant to sexual health, one needs look no further than the HIV/AIDS epidemic of the 1980s and 1990s. Originally termed gay-related immune deficiency (GRID) and thought to be an exclusively 'gay disease', the emergence of HIV/AIDS brought with it the increased stigmatization of gay and bisexual men as well as that of men who have sex with men (MSM; [13])—a stigma, which is still pervasive in certain parts of the world today [14].[2] Further expanding upon such experiences of discrimination, in their report on LGBT older adults' health, Fredriksen-Goldsen et al. [16] found that 82% of older LGBT adults had been victimized at least once on account of their perceived sexual orientation and/or gender identity and that internalized stigmatization got worse for LGBT adults the older they were—a likely result of older SGMs having lived in a time when their sexual orientation and/or gender identity had comparatively less societal acceptance and was even criminalized. For example, same-sex sexual behaviours in the Republic of Ireland were only decriminalized in 1993 [17]. In addition to 'obscuring' older SGM adults from population counts, this perceived discrimination may also have negative implications with regard to older LGBTQ+ adults' sexual health and functioning, as will be highlighted later in this chapter. However, this is not the only stigma that older LGBTQ+ adults experience with respect to their sexuality. Specifically, societal mores tend to desexualize older adults. For example, older adults are discouraged from discussing/expressing their sexuality [18]—it is almost as if older adults are expected not to be sexual at all. It is often only deemed appropriate for older adults to discuss sex and sexuality if it is done so in very specific ways; for example, it is deemed appropriate for older adults to make self-insulting ageist jokes about their lack of sex life and/or poor sexual functioning

---

[2] The AIDS epidemic of the 1980s and 1990s also resulted in the short- and long-term deaths of countless sexually active men who have sex with men [15], which may have resulted in a smaller number of older sexual minority men who are alive today.

[19]. Further complicating older adults' inability to discuss their sexuality, there is also a general infantilization of older adults that occurs within western societies [20]—a phenomenon that is perhaps best exemplified by the existence of 'elderspeak', a form of speech that is directed to older persons and which mimics 'babytalk' [21]. In turn, this general expectation that older adults should be treated like children and should not express their sexuality coupled with a lifelong history of LGBTQ+ specific stigmatization may have profound implications with regard to older SGM adults' willingness to openly express not only their sexual orientation and/or gender minority status but also their willingness and confidence to be open about their sexual needs, desires, and sexual health. As such, older SGM adults may not have been as likely to 'come out' in previous years as a result of increased stigmatization at the time and may not be as likely to 'come out' now that they are older due to stigmatization surrounding older adults' expressions of sex and sexuality. Indeed, findings demonstrate how older SGM adults are less likely to be open about their sexual orientation and/or gender identity than are younger adults [22]. In turn, this unwillingness on the part of older SGM adults to outwardly identify as LGBTQ+ partially impacts researchers' abilities to accurately determine the precise number of older adults who are LGBTQ+ or who engage in same-sex sexual activities and/or same-sex relationships. Thus, many more older adults may not actively be 'out' about their sexual orientation and/or gender identity than are actively reported, especially in certain parts of the world in which there are still laws that prohibit and punish acts of homosexuality [23, 24].

And yet, in spite of the large number of older adults who do not openly identify as LGBTQ+, as has already been stated, the number of older adults who do identify as SGMs is on the rise in the western world [1–3]. In particular, the number of older adults who openly identify as LGBTQ+ is being bolstered by those younger adults, who may be more likely to be open about their SGM status on account of temporal differences with regard to the acceptance of SGMs [22], and who are now ageing past 'middle age' and into 'young-old age'. Furthermore, the advent of treatment options for STIs like highly active antiretroviral therapy (HAART) for HIV/AIDS has resulted in more LGBTQ+ adults reaching old age in western countries where such treatment options are available and increasingly accessible via public healthcare systems [25]. As such, it seems logical to conclude that the number of older adults who openly identify as LGBTQ+ will continue to rise in the coming years.

Because of the increasing prevalence of older SGM adults in western societies, it has become exceedingly important for clinicians, medical professionals, care home residence workers, and others to hold a base understanding of older LGBTQ+ adults' sexual and gender identities as well as their sexual health and functioning. As much as society may deem it inappropriate to hear these facts discussed in the context of older adults, many older LGBTQ+ adults *are* still sexually active today [26–28]. Indeed, some studies have even highlighted how a majority of older gay men report wanting to have more frequent sex [29], and how older gay and bisexual men may be likely to have multiple sexual partners [26]. Further, it has been argued that concepts like 'lesbian bed death' (i.e., the idea that sexual frequency rapidly declines in lesbian relationships; [30]) are largely dated and non-factual [30–32].

Accordingly, given the prevalence and importance of LGBTQ+ older adults' sex lives, it is the purpose of this chapter to provide a succinct, yet comprehensive overview of the research that exists on older LGBTQ+ adults' sexual functioning and sexual health. While minimal research exists on this topic at present (see [33, 34]), the current research can be themed into three general categories, which will serve as the basis of this chapter: (1) the impact of SGM-related stigma and discrimination on older LGBTQ+ adults' willingness to 'come out' to healthcare workers and other related professionals, which, in turn, negatively affects their sexual functioning and health; (2) the relative risk of sexually transmitted infections (STIs) and other sex-related issues that older LGBTQ+ adults experience; and (3) older SGM adults' levels of sexual satisfaction. Following a discussion of these points, areas for future research will be provided, with emphasis placed on those specific domains, which feature a dearth of information.

6.1 The Impact of Stigma on Older LGBTQ+ Adults' Sexual Functioning and Health

As has already been stated, older LGBTQ+ adults experience stigmatization by virtue of their SGM status. In particular, this stigmatization may be compounded for gender minority individuals that occupy a visible minority status. For example, research has demonstrated how transgender persons report experiencing increased levels of prejudice and discrimination—a fact that researchers have attributed to a phenomenon called stigma visibility (i.e., 'the extent to which one holds a known, visible, conspicuous, and discredited stigmatized status'; [35], p. 812). Furthermore, transgender persons living in long-term care residences who require additional assistance with bodily functions and/or bathing may experience discrimination from workers on account of their inability to avoid disclosing their gender minority status [36]. In turn, the fear of discrimination that many older SGM adults feel may lead some of older LGBTQ+ adults to actively choose to avoid disclosing their sexual orientation and/or gender minority status to the relevant professionals. For instance, researchers have found that older sexual and gender minority adults living in long-term care homes are more likely to expect to experience discrimination from long-term care workers on account of negative past experiences, and that those older adults who expect this discrimination are less likely to be open with care workers about their SGM status ([37]; see [38], for a systematic review of those studies that have assessed LGBT persons' fears of discrimination in long-term care home settings). Indeed, additional research has highlighted how older gay and lesbian adults would prefer to live in 'gay-friendly' or gay 'exclusive' retirement homes [39]; alternatively, participants claimed that educating long-term care staff and residents—who also serve as a potential source of discrimination—about sexual and gender minority issues could serve to diminish discrimination in such facilities [39]. By electing to not disclose their LGBTQ+ status to care workers, older SGM adults run the risk of not having their sexual needs addressed; however, disclosing one's sexual orientation and/or gender minority status can also result in discrimination from long-term care workers, which may lead to SGM residents' sexual identities being ignored and their sexual health needs not being met [40].

In addition to long-term care workers, older LGBTQ+ adults may also choose to not disclose their SGM status to healthcare providers and medical professionals. Like with long-term care workers, this failure to disclose is often also the result of anticipated discrimination from healthcare professionals. To illustrate just how common nondisclosure is among older SGMs, in their recent study of 101 older LGB adults living in Lisbon, Portugal, Pereira et al. [28] found that 71.3% of participants had not disclosed their sexual minority status to their healthcare professionals, and that this was more common for women than for men. Similar findings with regard to gender were also reported by Gardner et al. [41] whose study showed that lesbian women were more fearful about 'coming out' than were gay men—a finding that the authors partially attributed to the accumulation of multiple minority stressors that older lesbian women face (see [42], for a discussion of minority stress). Returning to the idea of nondisclosure, Rosati et al. [43] similarly found that Italian sexual minority older adults were unwilling to disclose their sexual minority status unless they were interacting with a healthcare worker who they also knew to be another sexual minority person, or it was strictly necessary for them to disclose their SGM status in order to receive proper treatment. Results from the United States paint a similar picture, as well, with 21% of older LGBT adults not disclosing their sexual orientation to their general practitioner [44]. Specific national differences may play a role in rates of disclosure, as SGM identities are more accepted in certain parts of the world than others [23, 24]. Thus, overall, it would appear that older SGM individuals are either reluctant to disclose their minority status on account of a fear of discrimination from healthcare workers or that they are not actually asked to do so by their healthcare provider(s) [45]. Importantly, this latter point emphasizes the role that heterosexism plays in the disclosure process; that is, most patients are assumed by their medical professionals to be straight until *they* 'come out' on their own terms [46, 47] or their identity is inadvertently disclosed. Brotman et al. [48] have highlighted how this lack of disclosure is the likely result of a distrust with healthcare professionals on the part of SGM persons, as the healthcare system has historically attempted to 'cure' or 'fix' LGBTQ+ individuals. The role of heterosexism is further compounded by traditional conceptualisations of sex as occurring in monogamous dyads and primarily serving procreative purposes.

Demonstrating why SGMs are fearful of disclosing their sexual and/or gender minority status to healthcare workers, when older LGBTQ+ people do 'come out' to healthcare professionals about their SGM status, there is the potential that they will experience increased levels of discrimination and prejudice. For instance, according to Sharek et al. [49], less than half of older LGBT adults (43%) living in Ireland reported feeling that their healthcare professionals actively respected their LGBT status. Similar findings, which emphasize experiences of discrimination by healthcare professionals, have also been presented in a study of qualitative semi-structured interviews of older Canadian LGBT adults (some of whom were HIV positive):

I remember the doctor telling, 'I don't deal with people like you, you're HIV+, there's a place that you need to go, and this is it.' And I felt alone, depressed, didn't have the resources until I was connected and I went to Dr. [redacted] and the amazing clinic, but to be told that was like heart-breaking. Totally awful. (Participant quote from [50], p. 27)

At its worst, this fear of discrimination from healthcare professionals may be so salient that it leads some older LGBTQ+ adults to avoid seeking healthcare options altogether. For example, findings from a survey of 6502 LGBTQ adults living in the southern United States revealed that almost half of participants avoided accessing treatment options on account of discrimination previously experienced from healthcare workers ([51]; see also [52]). Thus, it would appear that older LGBTQ+ individuals are faced with a difficult choice: (1) they may choose to avoid treatment altogether and thereby avoid discrimination; (2) they may elect to 'come out' to their healthcare providers and hope that they are not discriminated against on account of their SGM status; or (3) they may decide to seek treatment while not disclosing their LGBTQ+ identity to their healthcare professionals and hope that they still receive adequate and appropriate treatment.

While electing to not disclose one's SGM status to healthcare professionals may potentially alleviate experiences of discrimination and prejudice, failure to do so can also have deleterious effects, especially if those minority statuses are directly related to medical concerns that would otherwise be addressed [53]. Specifically, physicians may not know what healthcare options are best for their patients without knowledge of their patients' SGM status and, by extension, their patients' sexual practices. For instance, healthcare providers may not know to recommend pre-exposure prophylaxis (PrEP) to their male patients who have sex with men as a preventative measure against HIV/AIDS if they are unaware of their patients' status as MSM [54]. Adding to the issues surrounding a lack of patient education, there is also an absence of sex-related programming specifically designed for older LGBTQ+ adults. For example, Hillman [55] has highlighted how there is a need for specific HIV/AIDS education programming for older LGBT adults living in the United States. In large part, this lack of formal education opportunities is the result of a dearth of research, which is specific to older LGBTQ+ adults more generally. Indeed, most sex-related research on older adults assumes heterosexual monogamy [56]; which, in turn, ignores older SGMs, while, at the same time, highlighting stereotypes surrounding older adults (i.e., that older adults *must* be heterosexual). Thus, taken together, older LGBTQ+ individuals may be less likely to be aware of their options with regard to sexual health and functioning than are older heterosexual individuals for whom research, and practice guidelines, are more prevalent; in turn, and as will be highlighted later in this chapter, this may lead to unnecessary health complications that would otherwise be avoidable.

Acting to further complicate matters for older LGBTQ+ adults' sexual health and functioning, medical diagnoses also tend to stigmatize SGM individuals in that such definitions are often also heterosexist. For instance, definitions of erectile dysfunction (ED) are centred around vaginal penetrative sex and do not take into account other forms of sex, which may be more common among certain SGMs [57].

In particular, men who exclusively have sex with men do not engage in vaginal penetrative sex, instead tending to engage in anal and oral sex with another man, neither of which are properly accounted for by ED definitions. Further, traditional definitions of ED do not fully take into consideration the erectile capacities of those men who are not 'active players' in the sex process (e.g., those men who receive anal sex or who perform fellatio). Similar definitions also exist with regard to premature ejaculation (PE). Specifically, definitions of PE emphasize intravaginal sexual activity, which, as is the case for ED, does not fully take into account the experiences of MSM [58]. Related to the idea of heterosexist definitions, research on sexual disorders among older LGBTQ+ adults is also limited and tends to focus on cisgender heterosexual individuals. As an example, in their structured literature review of research conducted on prostate cancer among gay, bisexual, and other men who have sex with men (GBM) populations, Rosser et al. [59] found very few studies conducted on the topic with GBM populations in spite of the fact that prostate cancer is the most common type of cancer found among GBM persons. Thus, it would appear that LGBTQ+ older adults are inadvertently discriminated against by researchers vis-à-vis a lack of comprehensive research. In the following section, which focuses on the presence of STIs and other sex-related health concerns among older LGBTQ+ adults, some of the implications of this paucity will be highlighted.

6.2 STIs and Other Sex-Related Issues Among Older LGBTQ+ Adults

Much like with younger sexually active individuals, STIs also potentially pose a problem for older adults. However, STIs are often overlooked in older adult populations. For example, Tillman and Mark [60] highlight how the number of older adults with STIs is often underestimated. Demonstrating this, recommendations for safe sex practices are often worded such that they are specific to a younger population, thereby omitting older adults [60]. The U.S. Preventative Services Task Force [61], for instance, only recommends that persons between the ages of 15 and 65, as well as those who are at an increased risk level for STIs (i.e., those who have had unprotected anal or vaginal sex or who have had sex with a new partner), receive screening for HIV/AIDS.[3] Additionally, research also highlights how healthcare providers may dismiss or misdiagnose STIs like HIV/AIDS in older adults as signs of ageing [63]. Finally, upper age limits on national sexual health surveys are commonplace—a trend, which does not take into account the experiences of the oldest adults [60]. Thus, it would appear that Tillman and Mark [60] are correct in their assertions that STIs are often underestimated within older adult populations.

Problematically, STIs may also pose a greater risk for LGBTQ+ older adults. Indeed, studies have highlighted how older SGM individuals may be at a particularly high risk level for contracting/having already contracted specific STIs. For

---

[3] Some scholars have claimed that the definition of older adults with the "greatest social need" should be broadened to include LGBT elderly persons [62].

example, Simone et al. [64] found that older transgender women were at an increased risk for contracting HIV/AIDS (see also [65]). Similarly, MSM have been shown to be 27 times more likely to contract HIV/AIDS than heterosexual men [65]—a problem for both younger and older MSM. This latter point is not particularly surprising as HIV/AIDS was stereotyped as a 'gay disease' [13]. Apart from HIV/AIDS, women who have sex with women may also be at an elevated risk for contracting human papillomavirus (HPV); findings demonstrate how 20% of older adult women who have never had heterosexual intercourse, but who may have engaged in same-sex intercourse, still have HPV, which is one of the leading causes of cervical cancer [57]. Finally, research also generally suggests that SGM individuals experience elevated levels of broader sex-related problems. For instance, in comparison to heterosexual men, gay and bisexual men report having increased levels of sex-related anxiety, a loss of interest in sex, more experiences of non-pleasurable sex, a greater inability to climax, and elevated levels of ED [66]. Similar findings have also been found for transgender women. Specifically, trans women individuals who have undergone intestinal vaginoplasty as part of vaginal reconstructive surgery have been shown to potentially experience increased levels of subsequent dyspareunia (i.e., vaginal pain during sex). One review study, for instance, found that 24.7% of trans women who had undergone intestinal vaginoplasty experienced dyspareunia during subsequent sexual encounters [67]. Conversely, other studies have found that the rate of dyspareunia is much lower trans women, though. Neto et al. [68], for example, found that only 2% of patients whose sex was assigned as male at birth who subsequently underwent gender confirmation surgery went on to experience dyspareunia. It is worth noting, though, that the patients in Bouman et al.'s [67] study had undergone intestinal vaginoplasty, whereas the patients in Neto et al.'s [68] study had undergone penile inversion vaginoplasty. The use of distinct types of vaginoplasty may, in turn, have implications with respect to subsequent health outcomes like dyspareunia in trans women who have undergone gender confirmation procedures.

While there are any number of potential risk factors that may lead to elevated rates of STIs and other sexual-related problems among older LGBTQ+ adults, certain risk factors stand out as being particularly concerning. Principal among these reasons is a general lack of education about topics like STIs among older SGMs. For example, older trans persons reported how they tended to not utilize safe sex techniques after they first transitioned, on account of a lack of knowledge about the importance of such practices [69]. This, in turn, may have put them at an elevated risk of contracting STIs. Related to this, research has also demonstrated how a not insignificant proportion of gay and bisexual men lack information with respect to HIV/AIDS [28]—a serious problem given the increased risk of contracting the infection among MSM to begin with [65]. Worth noting here, as well, research conducted by Cottrell [70] emphasizes how it is important for more than just MSM to receive screening for STIs like HIV/AIDS; this may not be a known fact among particular SGM and non-SGM older adults, though, given the conflation of HIV/AIDS and sexual minority status [13]. Further problematizing matters, this general absence of education about STIs and other sex-related issues is often the result of the discrimination, which as has been previously described, many older LGBTQ+ adults receive from healthcare workers. Specifically, the fact that many older LGBTQ+ individuals do not seek out assistance from doctors with regard to sexual-related issues on account of the fear of discrimination (e.g., [28, 43, 44]) may lead to these individuals' having a greater paucity of information with regard to important sexual health-related topics. This, in turn, may have negative implications in that these individuals may not receive enough information about the prevention and treatment of STIs and other sexual health-related issues to be able to take proper recourse when they are faced with such problems. For example, LGBTQ+ adults may not be aware of, or may not be willing to request, preventative and post-contraction treatment options for HIV/AIDS, such as HAART, if they are not willing to disclose their SGM status, sexual practices, and/or symptoms to their doctor(s) in a timely manner.

And yet there are still other ways in which discrimination from the healthcare system can negatively influence older LGBTQ+ adults' knowledge levels about, and ability to act on, sexual health-related issues. Specifically, older LGBTQ+ adults may have a harder time obtaining health insurance in select (western) countries such as the United States. For instance, Hillman [57] and Dibble et al. [71] have emphasized how lesbian women are less likely to receive sufficient health insurance, which may, in turn, result in an increased risk of certain types of cancer. Related to this, transgender individuals may also lack health insurance [72] and, even in those cases where they are insured, be unable to receive gender reassignment surgery as quickly as they would like due to plans that do not cover such operations [73, 74]. Having health insurance has also been linked to positive outcomes in the form of increased knowledge of STIs, as well. For instance, Brunsberg et al. [75] found that MSM who had health insurance were 28% less likely to have had unprotected anal intercourse, which may have been connected to their lower rates of HIV/AIDS. Thus, given the available evidence, it would appear that a lack of knowledge surrounding sexual health coupled with a lack of access to treatment options may lead some older LGBTQ+ adults to experience sexual health-related problems including but not limited to STIs. In the following section, we discuss another aspect of sexual health and functioning that can also potentially be influenced by discrimination and prejudice; specifically, the next section focuses on LGBTQ+ older adults' relative levels of sexual satisfaction.

6.3 Sexual Satisfaction Among Older LGBTQ+ Adults

According to scholars, maintaining an active and satisfying sex life is extremely important for a majority of older adults [76]. Further, there are multiple different ways in which individuals can ensure that they are maintaining as fulfilling and satisfying a sex life as possible. For example, older adults have been shown to be the most content sexually when they frequently engage in sex [77], consistently reach orgasm during intercourse [78], and participate in a variety of different sexual activities [76]. Overall, findings are mixed with regard to older adults' experiences of sexual satisfaction. For instance, 40–60% of a sample of predominately heterosexual older European adults reported being sexually satisfied [79]. One group, in particular, that has the potential to be especially dissatisfied with their sex lives is older LGBTQ+ adults.

While research on the topic is generally limited (see [80]), those studies that do exist with regard to older LGBTQ+ persons' sexual satisfaction generally tend to paint a mixed picture. For instance, according to Grabovac et al. [1], LGB older adults living in England reported having significantly less satisfaction with their overall sex lives when compared to heterosexual older adults. Similarly, according to Gillespie [76], LGB older adults were more likely to report being less satisfied sexually than were their heterosexual counterparts; worth noting, Gillepsie [76] found these results in spite of the fact that all of the participants in their study were in long-term relationships (i.e., participants were either cohabiting with a partner or were married). Research conducted by Lyons et al. [29] with older Australian gay men, in contrast, demonstrates how 60-year-old gay men are just as satisfied sexually as are 40-year-old gay men. Similarly, studies on transgender individuals who have undergone gender confirmatory surgery have generally emphasized how participants are sexually satisfied following their sex reassignment operations [81, 82] and how sexual satisfaction is positively correlated with surgery outcomes like increased vaginal depth and increased clitoral sensitivity among trans women [82]. Worth noting, LeBreton et al. [82] also found that trans women were generally dissatisfied with their sex lives prior to undergoing vaginoplasty.

Studies have demonstrated how sexual dissatisfaction among LGBTQ+ older adults may be the result of factors, which are extraneous to the experience of sex itself. For instance, Grabovac et al. [1] highlight how older LGB adults' sexual satisfaction may be lower on account of unwanted social experiences such as rejection, ageism, and discrimination from others, which may lead to older LGB persons holding a more negative outlook on life (see also [83]). Similar findings are also presented by Gonçalves et al. [84], who found that older Portuguese gay and bisexual men were often less sexually satisfied if they felt the need to conceal their sexual identity and internalized their experiences of stigmatization. In direct contrast to this, research has also shown how certain factors can also contribute to LGBTQ+ older adults having higher levels of sexual satisfaction. Lyons et al. [29], for instance, found that sexual satisfaction was positively correlated with self-esteem and subjective well-being in older gay men. Similarly, Fleishman et al. [4] found that older adults in same-sex relationships generally had moderate levels of sexual satisfaction and that sexual satisfaction was positively correlated with relationship satisfaction. Thus, overall, given the limited literature, it would appear that LGBTQ+ older adults have the potential to lead both satisfying and dissatisfying sex lives and that their satisfaction levels may be influenced both positively and negatively by extraneous factors like relationship satisfaction and/or perceived discrimination.

Overall, and as has already been stated, there is a general lack of research concerning older LGBTQ+ adults' sexual satisfaction, though [80]. In part, this is the result of national surveys directed towards older gay men and lesbian women, which ignore bisexual and transgender persons [57]. Further emphasizing how trans populations are understudied in this regard, there is an assumption that medical intervention in the form of sex reassignment surgery is often necessary before transgender persons can experience sexual satisfaction [85]. Accordingly, few studies have actually sought to investigate transgender persons' levels of sexual satisfaction prior to medical intervention ([85]; c.f., [82]). Further highlighting the ways in which older LGBTQ+ adults' sexual satisfaction levels are often ignored by researchers, a large proportion of the surveys utilized emphasize rates of sexual activity among older LGBTQ+ adults rather than their actual levels of sexual satisfaction [57]. It is also worth noting how many of those studies that do attempt to assess SGMs sexual satisfaction are insufficient in that they have utilized measures, which have not been properly validated with LGBTQ+ populations. For instance, it has been shown that the Interpersonal Exchange Model of Sexual Satisfaction Questionnaire (IEMSSQ) is utilized in one fifth of studies on gay men's sexual satisfaction despite its not having been properly validated at the time (see [86], for a study that validates the IEMSSQ with gay men and lesbian women). Thus, taken together, it would appear that there is a need for increased research into older LGBTQ+ adults' sexual satisfaction. In the following section, the dearth of research that generally surrounds ageing SGMs' sexual health and functioning will be highlighted in more detail.

6.4 Areas for Future Research

Throughout this chapter, we have repeatedly highlighted the relative paucity of research that exists with respect to older LGBTQ+ adults' sexual health and functioning. For instance, Dai and Meyer [33] emphasize how there is a lack of research related to older LGBT peoples' general health, despite government initiatives designed to address such knowledge gaps. In addition, and more specifically to the topic at hand, Slack and Aziz [34] claim that available studies on sexual health and functioning tend to have a heteronormative focus in that they exclude LGBTQ older populations (see also [56]). Accordingly, there is a clear need for additional research on all of the aforementioned components of older LGBTQ+ adults' sexual health and functioning.

Moreover, much of the research that does exist with respect to older SGMs' sexual functioning and health tends to focus on specific LGBTQ+ subpopulations such as gay men and/or lesbian women. As has been highlighted throughout this chapter, few studies actually place focus on bisexual individuals or gender minority persons (see [57]). Further demonstrating this point, Fredriksen-Goldsen [16] highlighted out how their study was 'unique' in that it included a substantial sample of transgender older adults. Furthermore, and problematically, a majority of the studies highlighted throughout this chapter are also characterized by the use of homogenous samples. Specifically, despite these studies placing focus on LGBTQ+ individuals, many of the participants in these studies are also white, to the exclusion of people of colour and other ethnic minority populations. For example, in Rosati et al.'s [43] qualitative study of 23 Italian sexual minority older adults, 100% of participants were white. Kum [87] and Witten [69] highlight how older LGBTQ+ adults of colour may face additional racial and ethnic stressors (see [42], for a discussion of minority stress), and how additional research is desperately needed on the intersectionality between race/ethnicity, age, and SGM status. Accordingly, it would appear that there is a need to diversify our understanding of LGBTQ+ older adults with respect to sexual health and functioning, something which can be accomplished by including older SGMs of colour in future research studies.

6.5 Conclusion

The purpose of this chapter has been to synthesize and thematize research, which exists on older LGBTQ+ adults' sexual health and functioning. In general, there is a lack of research on this area. However, research that does exist on older LGBTQ+ adults' sexual health and functioning can be broken down into three general domains: (1) the role of stigmatization and discrimination in older SGMs' willingness to seek out treatment options related to sexual health; (2) the relative rate of STIs and other sex-related issues among LGBTQ+ older adults; and (3) older LGBTQ+ adults' levels of sexual satisfaction. In addition, there is one common theme that exists across all of these categories: experiences of discrimination. Specifically, expected discrimination has the potential to influence older LGBTQ+ adults' willingness to seek out treatment for their sexual health concerns, which may, in turn, lead to these individuals having an increased risk of certain STIs and other related sexual health issues. As well, internalized experiences of discrimination may contribute to older LGBTQ+ persons having less satisfying sex lives. Accordingly, additional research on older LGBTQ+ adults' sexual health and functioning should also take into account experiences of discrimination and stigmatization in order to obtain a fuller picture of such issues. Only through learning more about older SGMs' sexual health and functioning will health and care workers be able to properly address older LGBTQ+ adults' sexual needs.

References

1. Grabovac I, Smith L, McDermott DT, Stefanac S, Yang L, Veronese N, Jackson SR. Well-being among older gay and bisexual men and women in England: a cross-sectional population study. JAMDA. 2019;20(9):1080–5. https://doi.org/10.1016/j.jamda.2019.01.119.
2. Kottorp A, Johansson K, Aase P, Rosenberg L. Housing for ageing LGBTQ people in Sweden: a descriptive study of needs, preferences, and concerns. Scand J Occup Ther. 2016;23(5):337–46. https://doi.org/10.3109/11038128.2015.1115547.
3. Nowakowksi ACH, Chan AY, Miller JF, Sumeraru JE. Illness management in older lesbian, gay, bisexual, and transgender couples: a review. Gerontol Geriatr Med. 2019;5:1–10. https://doi.org/10.1177/2333721418822865.
4. Fleishman JM, Crane B, Koch PB. Correlates and predictors of sexual satisfaction for older adults in same-sex relationships. J Homosex. 2020;67(14):1974–98. https://doi.org/10.1080/00918369.2019.1618647.

5. LGBT Movement Advancement Project & Services and Advocacy for Gay, Lesbian, Bisexual and Transgender Elders. Improving the lives of LGBT older adults. LGBT Movement Advancement Project & Services and Advocacy for Gay, Lesbian, Bisexual and Transgender Elders. 2010.
6. Fredriksen-Goldsen KI, Kim H-J. The science of conducting research with LGBT older adults- an introduction to aging with pride: national health, aging, and sexual/gender study (NHAS). Gerontologist. 2017;57(S1):S1–S14. https://doi.org/10.1093/geront/gnw212.
7. Wilson T, Shalley F. Estimates of Australia's non-heterosexual population. Aust Popul Stud. 2018;2(1):26–38. https://doi.org/10.37970/aps.v2i1.23
8. Morrison TG, Katz JW, Mirzaei Y, Zare S. Body image and eating disorders among sexual and gender minority populations. In: Rothblum E, editor. The Oxford handbook of sexual and gender minority mental health. Oxford: Oxford University Press; 2020. p. 73–86.
9. Choi SK, Meyer IH. LGBT aging: a review of research findings, needs, and policy implications. Los Angeles, CA: The Williams Institute, UCLA School of Law; 2016.
10. Wilson K, Stinchcombe A, Kortes-Miller K, Enright J. Support needs of lesbian, gay, bisexual, and transgender older adults in the health and social environment. Counsell Spiritual. 2016;35(1):13–29. https://doi.org/10.2143/CS.35.1.3189089.
11. Hicks GR, Lee T-T. Public attitudes toward gays and lesbians: trends and predictors. J Homosex. 2006;51(2):57–77. https://doi.org/10.1300/J082v51n02_04.
12. Srinivasan S, Glover J, Tampi RR, Tampi DJ, Sewell DD. Sexuality and the older adult. Curr Psychiatry Rep. 2019;21:97. https://doi.org/10.1007/s11920-019-1090-4.
13. Herek GM, Capitanio JP. AIDS stigma and sexual prejudice. Am Behav Sci. 1999;42(7):1130–47. https://doi.org/10.1177/0002764299042007006.
14. Ferlatte O, Salway T, Oliffe JL, Trussler T. Stigma and suicide among gay and bisexual men living with HIV. AIDS Care. 2017;29(11):1346–50. https://doi.org/10.1080/09540121.2017.1290762.
15. Hogg RS, Strathdee SA, Craib KJP, O'Shaughnessy MV, Montaner JSG, Schechter MT. Modelling the impact of HIV disease on mortality in gay and bisexual men. Int J Epidemiol. 1997;26(3):657–61. https://doi.org/10.1093/ije/26.3.657.
16. Fredriksen-Goldsen KI, Kim HJ, Emlet CA, Muraco A, Erosheva EA, Hoy-Ellis CP, Goldsen J, Petry H. The aging and health report: disparities experienced among lesbian, gay, bisexual, and transgender older adults. Caring and aging with pride. 2011.
17. Ryan F. 'We'll have what They're Having': sexual minorities and the Law in the Republic of Ireland. In: Leane M, Kiley E, editors. Sexualities and Irish society: a reader. Dublin: Orpen Press; 2014.
18. Nyanzi S. Ambivalence surrounding elderly widows' sexuality in urban Uganda. Ageing Int. 2011;36(3):278–400. https://doi.org/10.1007/s12126-011-9115-2.
19. Nimrod G, Berdychevsky L. Laughing off the stereotypes: age and aging in seniors' online sex-related humor. Gerontologist. 2018;58(5):960–9. https://doi.org/10.1093/geront/gnx032.
20. McLafferty I, Morrison F. Attitudes towards hospitalized older adults. J Adv Nurs. 2004;47(4):446–53. https://doi.org/10.1111/j.1365-2648.2004.03122.x.
21. Corwin AI. Overcoming elderspeak: a qualitative study of three alternatives. Gerontologist. 2018;58(4):724–9. https://doi.org/10.1093/geront/gnx009.
22. Gates GJ. In U.S., more adults identifying as LGBT [data set]. Gallup [distributer]. 2017. https://news.gallup.com/poll/201731/lgbt-identification-rises.aspx.
23. Al-Abbas LS, Haider AS. The representation of homosexuals in Arabic-language news outlets. Equal Divers Inclusion. 2020;40(3):309–37. https://doi.org/10.1108/EDI-05-2020-0130.
24. Joint United Nations Programme on HIV and AIDS. UNAIDS data 2018. 2018. http://www.unaids.org/en/resources/2018/unaids-data-2018.
25. Lyons A, Pitts M, Grierson J, Thorpe R, Power J. Ageing with HIV: health and psychological well-being of older gay men. AIDS Care. 2010;22(10):1236–44. https://doi.org/10.1080/09540121003668086.

26. Goddard SL, Poynten IM, Petoumenous K, Jin F, Hillman RJ, Law C, Roberts JM, Fairley CK, Garland SM, Grulich AE, Templeton DJ. Prevalence, incidence and predictors of anal *chlamydia trachomatis*, and *Neisseria gonorrhoeae* and syphilis among older gay and bisexual men in the longitudinal study for the prevention of anal cancer (SPANC). Sex Transm Infect. 2019;95(7):477–83. https://doi.org/10.1136/sextrans-2019-054011.
27. Lindau ST, Schumm LP, Laumann EO, Levinson W, O'Muircheartaigh CA, Waite LJ. A study of sexuality and health among older adults in the United States. N Engl J Med. 2007;357(8):762–74. https://doi.org/10.1056/NEJMoa067423.
28. Pereira J, de Vries B, Serzedelo A, Serrano JP, Afonso RM, Esgalhado G, Monteiro S. Growing older out of the closet: a descriptive study of folder LGB persons living in Portugal. Int J Aging Hum Dev. 2019;88(4):422–39. https://doi.org/10.1177/0091415019836107.
29. Lyons A, Pitts M, Grierson J. Growing old as a gay man: psychosocial Well-being of a sexual minority. Res Aging. 2013;35(3):275–95. https://doi.org/10.1177/0164027512445055.
30. Iasenza S. Beyond "lesbian bed death": the passion and play in lesbian relationships. J Lesbian Stud. 2002;6(1):111–20. https://doi.org/10.1300/J155v06n01_10.
31. Cohen JN, Byers ES. Beyond lesbian bed death: enhancing our understanding of the sexuality of sexual-minority women in relationships. J Sex Res. 2014;51(8):893–903. https://doi.org/10.1080/00224499.2013.795924.
32. Nichols M. Lesbian sexuality/female sexuality: rethinking "lesbian bed death". Sex Relatsh Ther. 2004;19(4):363–71. https://doi.org/10.1080/14681990412331298036.
33. Dai H, Meyer IH. A population study of health status among sexual minority older adults in select U.S. geographic regions. Health Educ Behav. 2019;46(3):426–35. https://doi.org/10.1177/1090198188818240.
34. Slack P, Aziz VM. Sexuality and sexual dysfunctions in older people: a forgotten problem. BJPsych Adv. 2020;26(3):173–82. https://doi.org/10.1192/bja.2019.80.
35. Miller LR, Grollman EA. The social costs of gender nonconformity for transgender adults: implications for discrimination and health. Sociol Forum. 2015;30(3):809–31.
36. Brotman S, Ferrer I, Sussman T, Ryan B, Richard B. Access and equity in the design and delivery of health and social care to LGBTQ seniors: a Canadian perspective. In: Orel N, Fruhauf C, editors. Lesbian, gay, bisexual and transgender older adults and their families: current research and clinical applications. Washington, DC: American Psychological Association; 2015. p. 111–40.
37. Jackson NC, Johnson MJ, Roberts R. The potential impact of discrimination fears of older gays, lesbians, bisexuals and transgender individuals living in small- to moderate-sized cities on long-term health care. J Homosex. 2008;54(3):325–39. https://doi.org/10.1080/00918360801982298.
38. Caceres BA, Travers J, Primiano JE, Luscombe RE, Dorsen C. Provider and LGBT individuals' perspectives on LGBT issues in long-term care: a systematic review. Gerontologist. 2020;60(3):e169–1183. https://doi.org/10.1093/geront/gnz012.
39. Johnson MJ, Jackson NC, Arnette JK, Koffman SD. Gay and lesbian perceptions of discrimination in retirement care facilities. J Homosex. 2005;49(2):83–102. https://doi.org/10.1300/J082v49n02_05.
40. Stinchcombe A, Smallbone J, Wilson K, Kortes-Miller K. Healthcare and end-of-life needs of lesbian, gay, bisexual, and transgender (LGBT) older adults: a scoping review. Geriatrics. 2017;2(1):13. https://doi.org/10.3390/geriatrics2010013.
41. Gardner AT, de Vries B, Mockus DS. Aging out in the desert: disclosure, acceptance, and service use among midlife and older lesbians and gay men. J Homosex. 2014;61(1):129–44. https://doi.org/10.1080/00918369.2013.835240.
42. Meyer IH. Prejudice, social stress, and mental health in lesbian, gay, and bisexual populations: conceptual issues and research evidence. Psychol Bull. 2003;129(5):674–97. https://doi.org/10.1037/0033-2909.129.5.674.
43. Rosati F, Pistella J, Baiocco R. Italian sexual minority older adults in healthcare services: identities, discriminations, and competencies. Sex Res Social Policy. 2021;18(6):64–74. https://doi.org/10.1007/s13178-020-00443-z.

44. Fredriksen-Goldsen K. Resilience and disparities among lesbian, gay, bisexual, and transgender older adults. Public Policy Aging Rep. 2011;21(3):3–7. https://doi.org/10.1093/ppar/21.3.3.
45. Boehmer U, Case P. Physicians don't ask, sometimes patients tell: disclosure of sexual orientation among women with breast carcinoma. Cancer. 2004;101(8):1882–9. https://doi.org/10.1002/cncr.20563.
46. Arbeit MR, Fisher CB, Macapagal K, Mustanski B. Bisexual invisibility and the sexual health needs of adolescent girls. LGBT Health. 2016;3(5):342–9. https://doi.org/10.1089/lgbt.2016.0035.
47. Foglia MB, Fredriksen-Goldsen KI. Health disparities among LGBT older adults and the role of nonconscious bias. Hastings Cent Rep. 2014;44(s4):S40–4. https://doi.org/10.1002/hast.369.
48. Brotman S, Ryan B, Jalbert Y, Rowe B. The impact of coming out on health and health care access: the experiences of gay, lesbian, bisexual and two-spirit people. J Health Soc Policy. 2002;15(1):1–29. https://doi.org/10.1300/J045v15n01_01.
49. Sharek DB, McCann E, Sheerin F, Glacken M, Higgins A. Older LGBT people's experiences and concerns with healthcare professionals and services in Ireland. Int J Older People Nurs. 2015;10(3):230–40. https://doi.org/10.1111/opn.12078.
50. Wilson K, Kortes-Miller K, Stinchcombe A. Staying out of the closet: LGBT older adults' hopes and fears in considering end-of-life. Can J Aging. 2018;37(1):27–31. https://doi.org/10.1017/S0714980817000514.
51. Roemerman RM, Wright ER, Simpkins J, Saint MJ, LaBoy A, Shelby R, Andrews C, Higbee M. Southern survey key findings: conditions and life experiences of LGBTQ southerners. Atlanta, GA: National Center for Civil and Human Rights LGBTQ Institute; 2018. https://www.lgbtqsouthernsurvey.org/general-findings-report.
52. Westwood S, Willis P, Fish J, Hafford-Letchfield T, Semlyen J, King A, Beach B, Almack K, Kneale D, Toze M, Becares L. Older LGBT+ health inequalities in the UK: setting a research agenda. J Epidemiol Community Health. 2020;74(5):408–11. https://doi.org/10.1136/jech-2019-213068.
53. American Medical Association. AMA policy regarding sexual orientation: H-65.973 health care disparities in same-sex partner households. Chicago, IL: American Medical Association; 2009. https://www.ama-assn.org/ama/pub/aboutama/our-people/member-groups-sections/glbtadvisory-committee/ama-policy-regarding-sexual-orientation.page.
54. Qiao S, Zhou G, Li X. Disclosure of same-sex behaviors to health-care providers and uptake of HIV testing for men who have sex with men: a systematic review. Am J Mens Health. 2018;12(5):1197–214. https://doi.org/10.1177/1557988318784149.
55. Hillman J. Sexuality and aging: clinical perspectives. Berlin: Springer; 2012.
56. Asencio M, Blank T, Descartes L, Crawford A. The prospect of prostate cancer: a challenge for gay men's sexualities as they age. Sex Res Social Policy. 2009;6(4):38–51. https://doi.org/10.1525/srsp.2009.6.4.38.
57. Hillman J. The sexuality and sexual health of LGBT elders. In: Hash KM, Rogers A, editors. Annual review of gerontology and geriatrics. Berlin: Springer; 2017. p. 13–26.
58. Althof SE, Abdo CHN, Dean J, Hackett G, McCabe M, McMahon CG, Rosen RC, Sadovsky R, Waldinger M, Becher E, Broderick GA, Buvat J, Goldstein I, El-Meliegy AI, Giuliano F, Hellstrom WJG, Incrocci L, Jannini EA, Park K, et al. International society for sexual medicine's guidelines for the diagnosis and treatment of premature ejaculation. J Sex Med. 2010;7(9):2947–69. https://doi.org/10.1111/j.1743-6109.2010.01975.x.
59. Rosser BRS, Merengwa E, Capistrant BD, Iantaffi A, Kilian G, Kohil N, Konety BR, Mitteldorf D, Westm W. Prostate cancer in gay, bisexual, and other men who have sex with men: a review. LGBT Health. 2016;3(1):32–41. https://doi.org/10.1089/lgbt.2015.0092.
60. Tillman JL, Mark HD. HIV and STI testing in older adults: an integrative review. J Clin Nurs. 2015;24(15–16):2074–95. https://doi.org/10.1111/jocn.12797.
61. U.S. Preventative Services Task Force. Screening for HIV, topic page. 2013. http://www.uspreventativeservicestask-force.org/uspstf/upshivi.htm.

62. Cahill S, Valadéz R. Growing older with HIV/AIDS: new public health challenges. Am J Public Health. 2013;103(3):e7–e15. https://doi.org/10.2105/AJPH.2012.301161.
63. Wooten-Bielski K. HIV & AIDS in older adults. Geriatr Nurs. 1999;20(5):268–72. https://doi.org/10.1016/S0197-4572(99)70026-1.
64. Simone M, Meyer H, Eskildsen M, Appelbaum J. Caring for LGBT older adults. In: Makadon H, Mayer K, Potter J, Goldhammer H, editors. Fenway guide to lesbian, gay, bisexual, and transgender health. 2nd ed. Philadelphia, PA: American College of Physicians; 2015.
65. Joint United Nations Programme on HIV and AIDS. UNAIDS fact sheet 2018. 2018b. http://www.unaids.org/en/resources/fact-sheet.
66. Brennan-Ing M, Kaufman JE, Larson B, Gamarel KE, Seidel L, Karpiak SE. Sexual health among lesbian, gay, bisexual, and heterosexual older adults: an exploratory analysis. Clin Gerontol. 2020:1–13. https://doi.org/10.1080/07317115.2020.1846103.
67. Bouman M-B, van Zeijl MCT, Buncamper ME, Meikerink WJHJ, van Bodegraven AA, Mullender MG. Intestinal vaginoplasty revisited: a review of surgical techniques, complications, and sexual function. J Sex Med. 2014;11(7):1835–47. https://doi.org/10.1111/jsm.12538.
68. Neto RR, Hintz F, Rübben H, vom Dorp, F. Gender reassignment surgery—a 13 year review of surgical outcomes. Int Braz J Urol. 2012;38(1):97–107. https://doi.org/10.1590/s1677-55382012000100014.
69. Witten TM. Health and well-being of transgender elders. In: Hash KM, Rogers A, editors. Annual review of gerontology and geriatrics. Berlin: Springer; 2017. p. 27–41.
70. Cottrell DB. Considering the needs of older sexual and gender minority people. J Nurse Pract. 2020;16(2):146–50. https://doi.org/10.1016/j.nurpra.2019.11.013.
71. Dibble SL, Roberts SA, Nussey B. Comparing breast cancer risk between lesbians and their heterosexual sisters. Womens Health Issues. 2004;14(2):60–8. https://doi.org/10.1016/j.whi.2004.03.004.
72. Safer JD, Coleman E, Feldman J, Garofalo R, Hembree W, Radix A, Sevelius J. Barriers to health care for transgender individuals. Curr Opin Endocrinol Diabetes Obes. 2016;23(2):168–71. https://doi.org/10.1097/MED.0000000000000227.
73. Haber D. Gay aging. Gerontol Geriatr Educ. 2009;30(3):267–80. https://doi.org/10.1080/02701960903133554.
74. Institute of Medicine. The health of lesbian, gay, bisexual, and transgender people: building a foundation for better understanding. Washington, DC: National Academy Press; 2011.
75. Brunsberg SA, Rosser BRS, Smolenski D. HIV sexual risk behavior and health insurance coverage in men who have sex with men. Sex Res Social Policy. 2012;9(2):125–31. https://doi.org/10.1007/s13178-012-0085-2.
76. Gillespie BJ. Correlates of sex frequency and sexual satisfaction among partnered older adults. J Sex Marital Ther. 2017;43(5):403–23. https://doi.org/10.1080/0092623X.2016.1176608.
77. Kim O, Jeon HO. Gender differences in factors influencing sexual satisfaction in Korean older adults. Arch Gerontol Geriatr. 2013;56(2):321–6. https://doi.org/10.1016/j.archger.2012.10.009.
78. Penhollow TM, Young M, Denny G. Predictors of quality of life, sexual intercourse, and sexual satisfaction among active older adults. Am J Health Educ. 2009;40(1):14–22. https://doi.org/10.1080/19325037.2009.10599074.
79. Træen B, Štulhofer A, Janssen E, Carvalheira AA, Hald GM, Lange T, Graham C. Sexual activity and sexual satisfaction among older adults in four European countries. Arch Sex Behav. 2019;48(3):815–29. https://doi.org/10.1007/s10508-018-1256-x.
80. de Vries B. LGBT couples in later life: a study in diversity. Generations. 2007;31(3):18–23.
81. Klein C, Gorzalka BB. Continuing medical education: sexual functioning in transsexuals following hormone therapy and genital surgery: a review (CME). J Sex Med. 2009;6(11):2922–39. https://doi.org/10.1111/j.1743-6109.2009.01370.x.
82. LeBreton M, Courtois F, Journel NM, Beaulieu-Prévost D, Bélanger M, Ruffion A, Terrier J-E. Genital sensory detection thresholds and patient satisfaction with vaginoplasty in male-to-female transgender women. J Sex Med. 2017;14(2):274–81. https://doi.org/10.1016/j.jsxm.2016.12.005.

83. Wight RG, LeBlanc AJ, de Vries B, Detels R. Stress and mental health among midlife and older gay-identified men. Am J Public Health. 2012;102(3):503–10. https://doi.org/10.2105/AJPH.2011.300384.
84. Gonçalves JAR, Costa PA, Leal I. Minority stress in older Portuguese gay and bisexual men and its impact on sexual and relationship satisfaction. Sex Res Social Policy. 2020;17(2):209–18. https://doi.org/10.1007/s13178-019-00385-1.
85. Lindley L, Anzani A, Prunas A, Galupo MP. Sexual satisfaction in trans masculine and nonbinary individuals: a qualitative investigation. J Sex Res. 2021;58(2):222–34. https://doi.org/10.1080/00224499.2020.1799317.
86. Calvillo C, Sánchez-Fuentes MM, Parrón-Carreño T, Sierra JC. Validation of the interpersonal exchange model of sexual satisfaction questionnaire in adults with a same-sex partner. Int J Clin Health Psychol. 2020;20(2):140–50. https://doi.org/10.1016/j.jchp/2019.07.005.
87. Kum S. Gay, gray, black, and blue: an examination of some of the challenges faced by older LGBTQ people of color. J Gay Lesbian Mental Health. 2017;21(3):228–39. https://doi.org/10.1080/19359705.2017.1320742.

Risky Sexual Activity and Its Impact on Mental and Physical Health in Older Adults

Daragh T. McDermott and Igor Grabovac

7.1 Introduction

Physical and emotional intimacy, including sexual activities, are important components and ways in which people show their affection throughout their lives. Research suggests that a large proportion of older adults remain sexually active well into their older age, usually contradicting the common fallacy of celibacy or asexuality in older age (for more information on the prevalence of sexual activities in older adults, please see Chap. 2 of this book). With technological and pharmaceutical advancements, many of the age-related physiological changes that used to present an obstacle to having and maintaining an enjoyable sex life among the elderly are addressable and no longer present as significant challenges, particularly for men. However, this change brings with it a variety of additional issues, for which healthcare providers, public health professionals and healthcare systems in general may not have appropriately planned for or developed services to support. This includes older adults engaging in risky sexual behaviours and the associated health outcomes of such behaviour such as increased vulnerability to sexually transmitted infections (STIs) and their physical and psychological impacts. Given the considerable contribution that STIs have on the global disease burden, understanding the reasons for this vulnerability is of great importance to public health and health and social systems worldwide.

The largest issue confronted by epidemiologists and other researchers examining risky sexual activities in older adults is the overall lack and heterogeneity of

D. T. McDermott (✉)
NTU Psychology, School of Social Sciences, Nottingham Trent University, Nottingham, UK
e-mail: daragh.mcdermott@ntu.ac.uk

I. Grabovac
Department of Social and Preventive Medicine, Center for Public Health, Medical University of Vienna, Vienna, Austria
e-mail: igor.grabovac@meduniwien.ac.at

published literature and available evidence, which mirrors the seemingly low interest of healthcare providers in meaningfully engaging with older adults on issues of sex and sexuality. This is coupled with a failure to routinely assess the prevalence of sexual activities and behaviours in this population [1]. Furthermore, this paucity of literature is attributable to a seeming lack of understanding and recognition, by various public health policy makers and researchers, that older adults continue to express themselves sexually. Instead, it is wrongly assumed that sexuality and issues concerning risky sexual behaviour are somehow reserved for the youth, young and middle-aged adult populations. For example, the World Health Organization continues to routinely report data on the prevalence of human immunodeficiency virus (HIV) among adults up to 49 years of age [2]. Many national questionnaires on sexual health do not provide stratified data among respondents beyond 45 years of age and only in recent iterations has the UK National Survey on Sexual Attitudes and Lifestyle begun to extend their cut-off age beyond 44 years [3]. Furthermore, Levy et al. reported that 73% of all clinical trials aiming at the risk reduction associated with STIs excluded people over the age of 50 and 89% excluded participants over the age of 65 years [4].

However, of the sparse literature that is available, there is evidence that does indicate that older adults have increased vulnerability to STIs and overall demonstrate higher engagement in risky sexual behaviours. These may be the result of biological and physiological changes but are also linked to various social and psychological factors as well as a range of systemic factors. In this chapter we will outline the available data on engagement in risky sexual behaviour, present reasons for the increased vulnerability of older adults for STIs and provide an overview of how the impact of risky sexual behaviours influence health outcomes in general among older adult populations. Finally, we will identify a range of suggested ideas as to how healthcare providers can meaningfully engage with such topics with their older adult patients and clientele (for more information on this, see Chap. 12).

7.1.1 Defining Risky Sexual Behaviour

Defining "high-risk sexual behaviour" or "risky sexual activities" is difficult as most authors focus on reporting proportions or trends of activities regarded as falling in these categories without providing clear and succinct definitions. This is also by no means an easy feat, as these behaviours are heavily dependent on the context in which they occur with this being compounded by the additional challenge of the underreporting of these behaviours. On the one hand, many people may feel shame and may not be forthcoming about their sexual experiences, particularly if the prevailing perceptions are that people in this group are not expected to be sexually active and in circumstances where healthcare providers are reluctant or fail to ask the necessary questions regarding this topic. During epidemiological surveys, even if the questions are asked, participants tend to provide only socially desirable answers, which skew the data, which is especially true in older adults. Sexual behaviour includes a range of physical and emotional activities that gratify an individual's sexual needs, as such they have been studied in the context of sexual activities, practices, emotional relationships, transmission of sexually transmitted infections and unwanted pregnancies. Importantly, expression of sexuality is a normative phenomenon; however within prevailing cultural contexts, different behaviours or activities are questioned and/or deemed "risky" (which may be equated with the term high-risk sexual behaviour) [5]. Generally, in the medical field as well as within public health, most questions regarding human sexuality have focused on either reproduction or transmission of sexually transmitted infections; therefore most researchers define high-risk sexual behaviour as that which may increase risk of exposure among individuals to contracting an STI or resulting in unwanted pregnancies. As such, this further influences their health outcomes and in part explains why most available academic literature has focused on unprotected sexual intercourse or involvement in sexual activities with multiple partners [5].

Further, substance use and related abuse disorders have often been associated with high-risk sexual behaviours, with studies often highlighting that alcohol consumption influences the decision-making abilities of those engaged in sexual activities while intoxicated. Sexual activities, while inebriated, can lead to risky sexual behaviour such as having unprotected intercourse or other risk-taking behaviours. Various theoretical models have been proposed to explain the reasons behind alcohol consumption and engagement in risky sexual behaviour, with the most common within the literature being the alcohol myopia theory, expectancy theory and cognitive escape theory. Details on each of these are beyond the scope of this chapter; however they postulate that after consuming alcohol, individuals tend to focus on social cues which are rewarding and, in that way, instigate thoughts of the pleasurable aspects of having sex while distancing the thoughts of potential negative consequences or impacts of risky sexual activities, overall reducing sexual inhibition [6–9]. While associations of the overall effects of alcohol consumption and engagement in risky sexual behaviour have been well documented, it remains unclear to what extent is this also true for older adults. Grabovac et al. analysing data from 1622 men and 2195 men older than 50 years participating in a nationally representative cohort in England reported that over an 8-year follow-up, binge drinking was positively associated with sexual activity, with the odds of being sexually active at follow-up 52% higher for men and 57% higher for women [10]. Another study by Schick et al. reported that almost one quarter of men and 14% of women who are 50 years or older drank alcohol or had a partner who drank alcohol during their last episode of peno-vaginal intercourse [11].

Apart from use of alcohol, use of drugs (licit and illicit) in combination with sexual activities is receiving more and more attention from researchers. However, the vast majority of literature exploring this topic has focused mainly on gay and bisexual, and other men who have sex with men, within the confines of the so-called chemsex phenomenon. Emerging evidence indicates that a growing number of men and women, regardless of their sexual orientation, engage in use of drugs during sexual activities. As reported by Lawn et al. [12], in their analysis of the results of the Global Drug Survey, heterosexual as well as non-heterosexual men and women engaged in sex while under the influence of narcotic substances, with the most common (next to alcohol) being cannabis and 3,4-methylenedioxymethamphetamine (MDMA) and mostly attributable to their desire to "enhance sex". While the authors did report larger proportions of bisexual and gay men and women, they did show that in all groups more than 20% of participants reported having used drugs with the intent of enhancing sexual experiences. Further, in their conclusions, these authors noted that all men and women, irrespective of their sexual orientation or partner preference, should be considered when forming harm reduction and treatment strategies. Unfortunately, most evidence from this field of research again only focuses on the young or middle age adults (for example, in the study by Lawn et al., the mean age is reported around 31 years of age). There is some evidence to suggest that age may be a protective factor against the use of drugs for "sexual enhancement"; however this evidence is again limited to very specific subgroups such as men who have sex with men or people living with HIV [13, 14]. Due to this lack of evidence, more research in this area is warranted.

7.1.2 Engaging in Risky Sexual Behaviour in Older Adults

As discussed, there is a notable paucity of literature and evidence focused on sexually risky behaviour and sexual risk taking in older adults. A small number of studies have examined the knowledge and attitudes of older adults towards STIs, with most available literature focusing exclusively on their views and perceptions of HIV. In a 2015 study conducted among American Veterans aged over 60, using the "Knowledge of Sexually Transmitted Infections Survey", Jennings reported that mean levels of perceived knowledge of STIs were extremely low for all STIs: 1.84/5 for chlamydia, 1.94/5 for genital warts, 2.18/5 for gonorrhoea, 2.06/5 for hepatitis B, 2.24/5 for herpes, 2.69/5 for HIV/AIDS and 2.02/5 for syphilis [15]. Results in a larger survey of Australians older than 60, Lyons and colleagues analysed over 2000 participants who reported overall good general knowledge on STIs. However, concurrently, this same pool of participants reported poor knowledge in areas such as protection offered by condoms or the modes of transmission for STIs. Women as well as people who had previously been tested for STIs in general reported better overall knowledge scores [16]. With respect to HIV, older adults tended to have less knowledge regarding the transmission of HIV and the progression of the disease when compared to younger adults, with some studies reporting about a third of older adults demonstrated a complete lack of knowledge about HIV transmission. Zablotsky and Kennedy [17] reported that among women older than 50, 45% reported beliefs that HIV could be contracted through casual sexual encounters such as kissing. A study by Negin et al. [18] found that among a sample of 722 participants older than 50 years in sub-Saharan Africa, HIV knowledge was significantly lower than that of younger adults. Additionally, in the same sample, older adults were half as likely to be tested for HIV. Overall, this general lack of knowledge contributes to the misconceptions and inaccuracies associated with STI risk, which is continued by the fact that older adults consistently report few opportunities to talk about sexual health with their healthcare providers, thereby limiting appropriate access to educational resources and medical interventions [19, 20]. For example, Bergeron et al. reported that after turning 50, only about 24% of older women discussed sex with their healthcare provider. Similarly, data from a US study of over 3000 adults showed that only 38% of men and 22% of women between 57 and 85 years old discussed sex with a physician after the age of 50 [21].

Access to knowledge on preventive strategies has been demonstrated to influence engaging in safe sex; therefore, with evidence showing poor knowledge among older adults regarding safe sex and transmission of STIs, we can also presume that levels of protected sex practices to be low. This lack of knowledge is also compounded by the prevailing perception among older adults that they themselves are at no, or low, risk of contracting STIs. This has been demonstrated in a US data set collected from people older than 50 who received a positive HIV diagnosis, with most of them recorded as being without a known risk factor for contracting HIV. Rose [22] conducted a survey among people older than 60 regarding their knowledge and belief about HIV and AIDS. Most respondents were aware of AIDS being a serious illness but at the same time, most were not aware that they were also susceptible to contracting the virus. Therefore, it should not be surprising that evidence suggests overall use of sexual protection and contraception, such as condoms, among older adult populations is lower than other age groups. For example, even though a high proportion of older adults were found to have consumed alcohol or had a partner that had consumed alcohol during their last sexual encounter or episode of sexual intercourse, less than 25% reported having used a condom. This is despite more than 5% of the sample also revealing that their previous partner had been diagnosed with an STI. In the same study, the prevalence of condom use fluctuated as a function of "partner type" and age group. The highest percentages reported among men reporting condom use was with a "transactional partner" and women with a "friend"; however rates of use were still very low with reported levels only at 66.7% and 44.4%, respectively. With respect to condom use as a function of age, the highest prevalence of condom use during the last episode of intercourse was within 50–59-year age bracket, at 24.3%, with rates continuing to decline as age increased, with condom usage reported as being 17.1% among those 60–69 and 14.3% for those over the age of 80. Overall, prevalence of condom use in this study was recorded as being only 20% [11]. Further, a study by Cooperman et al., limited to men aged 49–80 years, reported that over the last 6 months only 18% of HIV negative and 58% of HIV positive men had used condoms consistently. In their foundational study, Lindau et al. used a national probability sample, which reported that more than 90% of men older than 50 years of age did not use condoms either with a date or a casual sexual partner. Concerningly, 70% reported that they did not use a condom when the partner was a stranger [21]. Evidentially, most of the aforementioned studies and results stem from research conducted in either the US of UK, with other countries, particularly those in the global south, being represented on a seldom basis, with data from Asian and African countries being especially scarce. However, of the data that is available, the situation seems to be similar or of greater concern. In a study of over 1700 individuals from the Chiang Mai region of Thailand, more than 90% of participants over the age of 30 reported not having used a condom during sexual intercourse in the preceding three months. Data were stratified by age and there was an unfortunate but consistent rise in the proportion of participants who had not used a condom by age category with the proportion being 94.2% in those 40–49 years old, 95.9% in 50–59 year olds and 98.1% in those over the age of 60 [23]. Similarly, results emerging from South Korea showed that in adults aged above 60 years old, 0% of respondents, male and female, reported regular condom use. Of this sample, the highest proportion (28.6%) of respondents reported "sometimes" (42.6% for males and 10.8% for females) using a condom with never using a condom being the most prevalent at 26.2% [24].

Concordant with the evidence on condom use, studies have noted that 90% of samples older than 50 do not get tested for HIV, with older women particularly being less likely to be tested for HIV when compared to younger women. Overall, the rates of HIV and STI tests are low in older adults. Data from Adekeye et al. showed that only 25% of American over the age of 50 had had an HIV test, and less than 4% plan to have another within the next year. Further research, by Schick et al., reported that 29.8% of men and 27.3% of women over the age of 50 were tested for HIV within the past year (with 38.6% and 32.5% never being tested). A similar result was found for other STI tests, where only 35.6% of men and 31.1% of women over the age of 50 had been tested for STIs within the past year. Promisingly, however, a UK-based study reported that the number of older women seeking help or support for the first time, in two sexual health clinics, quadrupled between 1998 and 2008 [25]. However, evidence on a pan-European basis is still lacking as there is currently no available data that allows for the aggregation of age groups after the age of 45 [26].

Despite the improvements of HIV therapy witnessed since the advent of the virus in the 1980s, emerging evidence highlights the rising incidence of HIV in older adults (see below). As such, it is imperative that we briefly outline available evidence concerning risky sexual behaviours among older adults who live with HIV. Studies here report differences between men and women, with men living with HIV being more commonly sexually active compared with women living with HIV. It should be noted that than 50% of both genders making a decision to completely stop engaging in partnered sexual activities. The most common reason for this decision is linked to high levels of stigma, fear, anxiety and rejection following a HIV+ disclosure. Among this population differences in condom use were also apparent; the lowest frequency was prevalent among gay and bisexual older men when compared to heterosexual peers. However, both male and female older adults living with HIV reported engaging in unprotected anal or vaginal intercourse [27]. This has been linked to the already mentioned, poor level of knowledge on protection and transmission of HIV but also to the lower levels of reliability of condoms when used by older men with various degrees of erectile dysfunction.

7.1.3 Sexually Transmitted Infections in Older Adults

Sexually transmitted infections (STIs), also referred to as sexually transmitted diseases (STDs), are infections that can be transmitted though oral, anal and vaginal sex. Overall, there are more than 30 different pathogens that may cause STIs, with eight of these being associated with the highest incidence of STIs on a global scale. Out of these eight identified, four are viral infections (hepatitis B, herpes simplex virus, HIV and human papillomavirus), three are bacterial (gonorrhoea, chlamydia and syphilis) and one is parasitic (trichomoniasis). All STIs are preventable; however only four are currently considered curable: syphilis, gonorrhoea, chlamydia and trichomoniasis. It is possible that a person has an STI, without presenting any symptomology; however most symptoms include vaginal or penile discharge, painful urination, genital ulcers and abdominal pain. For a more detailed overview on clinical presentation of STIs as well as their treatment please consult external sources.

STIs are among the most prevalent infections in human, with an estimated one million newly acquired infections daily. According to estimates from the WHO, in 2020 there have been more than 374 million new infections with one of the four STIs trichomoniasis being the most prevalent (with 156 million new cases), followed by chlamydia (129 million new cases), gonorrhoea (82 million new cases) and syphilis (7.1 million new cases). Additionally, in 2016, estimates were that around 300 million women worldwide had an HPV infection and 296 million people were living with a chronic hepatitis B infection (both infections being preventable with vaccination). The healthcare burden attributable to STIs goes beyond the consequences of the primary infection as some of these diseases increase the risk of contracting HIV (for example, herpes simplex infection, syphilis and gonorrhoea) or may cause cancer (as in HPV and cervical cancer and hepatitis B and hepatocellular carcinoma) [28].

Considering all this evidence, pointing to the significant public health concerns associated with STIs, data on their prevalence in older adults is seriously inadequate. As briefly mentioned in the introduction, rigorous epidemiological monitoring of STIs for groups of older adults is still largely unavailable. Therefore, limited available evidence on the trends of STI diagnoses in older adults stems from smaller cohorts or meta-analyses of studies of varying design and quality.

Overall, recent evidence highlights an increase in the rate of sexually transmitted infections, with the most prominent increases in diagnoses occurring in the younger age groups. Monitoring data from the United Kingdom stemming from reports of diagnoses in sexual health clinics showed that STI rates in the group of "45+" seem to be stable, despite reports of a first recorded increase in "ano-genital warts" among those 45–64 years old. A report of STI distribution of older adult patients visiting sexual health clinics in the West Midlands region of the UK showed that the rate of STIs in older adults doubled between 1996 and 2003. Levels increased from being 16.7 per 100.000 in 1996 to 36.3 per 100.000 in 2003. This trend was also observed for each of the selected infections including syphilis, gonorrhoea, chlamydia, ano-genital warts and herpes. Overall, men accounted for two thirds of the diagnoses. The authors of this study also noted that the most common route of infection was heterosexual transmission, with only 6% being accounted for same-sex transmission [29]. In Australia, it was noted that new diagnoses of gonorrhoea, chlamydia and syphilis had increased in those older than 50 between 2006 and 2010 [3]. Despite rates being lower than those in the younger population, a report from the USA demonstrated a rise in diagnosis rates of chlamydia in both men and women older than 55 between 2006 and 2010. Further, a study by Wang et al. reported 242.115 new syphilis diagnoses among older adults in the Guangdong region of China. This increase reflects a marked increase in the rate of diagnoses from 13.8 per 100.000 in 2004 to 112.0 per 100.000 population in 2019 (the average annual percent change being 16.5%). Finally, a study by Goddard et al., conducted in Australia, from data collected over a 36-month window, demonstrated an increase in the incidence of anal chlamydia, gonorrhoea and syphilis among older (35–79-year old) gay and bisexual men. During the 1428 person-years of follow-up (PYFU), the incidence per 100 PYFU was 10.40 for anal chlamydia, 9.11 for anal gonorrhoea and 5.47 for syphilis.

As iterated above, national and international monitoring of STI provides us limited data as most health agencies limit the collection of data and subsequent segregation of age groups in their reports. For example, when examining the reports on STI trends in Europe, published by the European Centre for Disease Prevention and Control (ECDC), data for older adults is only available as a 45+ group categorisation. However, an overall increase in this trend is visible with the proportion of new diagnoses of gonorrhoea in the 45+ age category rising from 5.3 per 100,000 in 2000 to 8.9 per 100,000 in 2010 and from 12.9 to 22.4 for syphilis during the same time frame [30]. In 2020, 21% of new HIV diagnoses were found in people over the age of 50, with more than 25% of new diagnoses in this age group being reported in Austria, Denmark, Finland, Luxembourg, Italy and the Netherlands. The most common route of HIV transmission in this age group is through unprotected heterosexual sex. These rates seem to be relatively stable in Europe [31]. However, Haddad reported an overall proportion of new HIV diagnoses in people older than 50 increased from 15.1% to 22.8% between 2008 and 2017, suggesting a worrying increase in transmissions. Rates have been steadily increasing for both men and women, with a relatively higher increase apparent among women. This trend was also reported by Mahy et al. [32], who analysed UNAIDS data in people aged over 50 years worldwide affirming the increasing trends in the prevalence of the virus. Despite these increases, however, pharmacological advances and improvements in therapy outcomes, including the inability to transmit the virus among those adhering to a post-exposure prophylaxis treatment plan and who have undetectable viral loads, as well as the recent rollout of pre-exposure prophylaxis (PREP), will hopefully mitigate against these increases and reduce the noted rise in virus transmissions. However, the primary target for many HIV awareness campaigns and the roll out of PREP has typically targeted men who have sex with men, gay and bisexual men and those considered clinically at risk. It is important that those responsible for such campaigns now include older populations and particularly older women in any ongoing or future interventions.

7.1.4 Older Adults and Vulnerability to Sexually Transmitted Infections

There are various reasons why older adults may be more susceptible to STIs compared to younger adults, and these may be biological and psychosocial in nature. In the following section, we will briefly outline some of the potential reasons as to why this may be the case.

7.1.4.1 Biological Issues

There are several physiological changes that occur across the lifespan and as people age, which may also affect the susceptibility of older adults to contracting STIs. Biologically, regardless of age, male-to-female transmission of HIV is more likely than female-to-male, which puts women under increased risks of HIV contraction regardless of the age group [33]. In addition, the lower levels of oestrogen that occur as a result of ageing and can coincide with the onset of the menopause may lead to less vaginal excretion during sex. The resulting vaginal dryness may lead to more micro-abrasions during sexual activity, which may facilitate the transmission of STIs [3]. Additionally, some studies have indicated that changes in the immunological milieu in the cervix may play an important role in HIV-1 transmission in heterosexual older women. It has been reported that CD4+ T cells in the cervix of older adult women had characteristics associated with elevated immune activation including expression of both CCR5 and CXCR4 chemokine receptors, which make it possible for HIV-1 to enter the cell. These results suggest that postmenopausal women may be at a greater risk of contracting HIV-1 compared to premenopausal women [34]. This is coupled with an apparent decline in the use of contraception, such as condoms, by this population group. In explanation for this, there is a sense that as postmenopausal women can no longer get pregnant, they do not use birth control to prevent unwanted pregnancies, which may lead to the erroneous perception that condoms are no longer as essential or useful as they were prior to the onset of menopause [35]. Older men tend not to demonstrate significant physiological changes that increase the predisposition for STIs; however as some men experience erectile dysfunction and among those that have undergone a prostatectomy, they may face urinary incontinence, which can lead to overall less consistency in using condoms or their correct usage [36].

7.1.4.2 Psychosocial Issues

Additionally, some studies suggest that many older people, particularly women, are involved in so-called self-silencing strategies and do not ask male partners about their risk-taking or risky sexual behaviours so as to avoid conflict [37]. Further, other studies have demonstrated that men are also reluctant to disclose their past risky sexual behaviours, including having engaged in unprotected sex with other men [38]. A literature review of studies investigating the prevalence of testing for STIs in older adults conducted by Savasta [39] noted that 88% of articles contained in their analysis focused on systemic health system issues, such as a lack of communication from healthcare providers and insufficient educational programmes.

Research has shown that older adults' vulnerability towards STIs may be based on this lack of appropriate avenues for seeking sexual health information and guidance. More alarming is the lack of materials on STIs and HIV that are specifically tailored to older adult populations. Given these difficulties in communication as well as findings that appropriate educational materials are lacking, it is speculated that older adults who have more social capital (i.e. higher socio-economic status and/or education) may have more access to information on safe sex, leading to less engaging in risky sexual behaviour, especially as social capital was associated with a variety of positive health outcomes in older adults. However, in a study by Amin [40], social capital was not found to be significantly associated with safe sex.

7.1.5 Health Outcomes Associated with Sexually Transmitted Infections in Older Adults

As established in this chapter, late presentation and recognition of sexually transmitted infections in older adults is common and may be associated with several etiological factors. The increased burden of STIs is primarily linked to late diagnosis, which brings about late initiation of treatment among these populations which can mean that care only commences at advanced stages of the disease, which can detrimentally impact recovery rates and increase the rate of complications. Additionally, delayed diagnosis of STIs increases the risk for transmission, as patients may unknowingly engage in risky sexual behaviour while being infectious themselves [29, 41]. With respect to syphilis, some studies report on an increasing trend towards diagnosis of the disease in the tertiary stage in older people, suggesting that many patients may have been living with the disease for considerable periods of time and due to the late onset of treatment did not receive an adequate or timely diagnosis. Tertiary syphilis can manifest as gummatous, cardiovascular or central nervous disease and increases the risk for acquiring and transmitting HIV, thus representing a significant additional factor to the morbidity of older adults [42]. As outlined previously, between 1995 and 2013, HIV prevalence doubled in patients aged 50 years or older [32], whilst a decreasing trend of HIV infection rates was observed in the population under 50 years of age [43]. In addition, progression from HIV infections to Acquired Immunodeficiency Syndrome (AIDS) was reported as significantly higher in older patients than in 25- to 29-year-olds [26]. Both findings may partly be due to late recognition and proper interpretation of symptoms by physicians, in part due to a lack of awareness or understanding on the part of physicians that older adults continue to maintain an active sex life and engage with multiple sex partners. The prolonging of the diagnostic process for HIV infections is of concern as delayed treatment greatly increases the risk of a person infecting others and risking health complications associated with the disease including the potential for progression to AIDS. Antiretroviral therapy (ART) is a treatment designed to supress viral replication and reduce the viral load in patients, with current treatment guidelines suggesting immediate initiation of therapy in order to achieve viral suppression [44]. Non-delaying ART is also important as proper treatment with ART reduces not only AIDS-associated mortality and morbidity but also reduces the risk for non-AIDS-related chronic diseases in people living with HIV (coronary, liver and kidney diseases, malignancies and neurologic disorders) [45]. A comparison of ART in patients aged 50 or older with a younger group revealed higher therapy adherence among the older population and accordingly lower viral loads [46, 47], but response rates to ART indicated by CD4 cell count were significantly slower in elderly patients [48]. These results suggest that, although the initial therapeutic benefit in older patients may be lower, high therapy adherence amongst the older populations still results in beneficial therapeutic outcomes. This is particularly important, as with the overall improvements in ART and prolonged survival of patients, the number of older HIV patients is expected to increase and may become a major public health concern [49].

7.1.6 Mental Health Outcomes Associated with Risky Sexual Behaviours in Older Adults

As previously noted, the literature associated with risky sexual behaviours in older adults is limited, in part attributable to the fallacy that older people are less likely to want to sustain an active sex life as they age. Despite this gap, there is a burgeoning set of literature that outlines the positive benefits of sustained sexual activity into later life. In a large cross-sectional study drawn from the English Longitudinal Study of Ageing involving near 6500 participants, L. Smith et al. [50] demonstrate that overall levels of well-being are higher among adults when they are engaged in sexual activities. Additionally, examinations of the effects of engaging in sexual activity in later life on both physical and mental health demonstrate associations with higher levels of motivations to engage in physical activity (e.g. walking), higher levels of social support, lower tobacco usage, use of fewer prescribed medications, engaging in social activities and overall greater psychological well-being [51].

However, this study does not indicate the extent to which the sexual behaviours that the respondents are engaged in are either classified as being safe sex or risky in nature with an evidence gap existing around the extent to which older adults are engaged in safe-sex behaviours. Of the available literature, a large-scale assessment by Foster et al. [52] showed that sexual self-efficacy was a key factor associated with older people's confidence in engaging in safer sex. This self-efficacy is influenced by participants' knowledge and awareness of sexual health issues. These findings are supported by work which explored both the socio-cultural and psychological factors associated with risky sexual behaviours. Their findings demonstrated that the propensity to engage in risky sexual behaviours can be explained by a lack of knowledge around sexual health matters, an increased perception of the importance of sex and for women, a lack of sexual self-efficacy and power in sexual decision making.

This is in part explained by the lack of relevant sexual health discussions between an older person and their physicians. Part of the reason why this gap is apparent may be explained by feelings of anxiety, guilt and shame on the part of the older person when speaking about sex and sexual activities due to cultural associations of sex and shame. In a qualitative study conducted with older adults, aimed at exploring reasons why people were reluctant to seek sexual health services, participants indicated that shame and embarrassment were a key factor as well as a sense that the increase in sexual difficulties or a decline in libido were all part of "normal ageing" [53]. An additional aspect cited by participants was an embarrassment of speaking about such topics with clinicians who were younger than them in age.

Taken together, these findings highlight that sexual activity among older adults is more common than might be assumed; however the extent to which the sex that is occurring is safe is questionable due to a lack of sufficient education and knowledge among these populations and the lack of relevant self-disclosure to their medical professionals. There is a clear need for healthcare providers to engage in open discussions about sex and sexual health with older people and to provide them with both clinical support for any sexual difficulties/dysfunctions that may emerge due to ageing, but also with the necessary sexual health information, such as the use of protection during sex, that can help mitigate against the spread of STDs. Further, there is a need for greater awareness by the full range of healthcare professionals, particularly those who work in residential community settings, around the benefits of sexual activity among the elderly, the importance of sexual health education and awareness for those engaged in sexual activity and the potential implications of unsafe sexual behaviours on long-term health outcomes.

7.2 Conclusion

Despite a paucity, increasing evidence demonstrates that there is a greater than previously observed level of sexual activity among the elderly. With this, there is a greater need for health professionals to be prepared to support older adults with their sexual health requirements. As demonstrated with our overview, levels of sexually transmitted infections are increasing among this demographic and this can have peripheral health impacts on a persons physical and mental health. There is a need on the part of medical professionals to be cognisant of older adult's sexual health and to be proactive in their discussion of these topics with their patients so as to help ameliorate growing levels of sexually transmitted infections among this population. Further, the potential benefits of sexual activity among the elderly should not be underestimated as increasing evidence suggests that sustained sexual activity has both physical and mental health benefits as people age.

References

1. Maes CA, Louis M. Nurse Practitioners' sexual history-taking practices with adults 50 and older. J Nurse Pract. 2011;7(3):216–22. https://doi.org/10.1016/j.nurpra.2010.06.003.
2. WHO. The Global Health Observatory: HIV/AIDS. 2021a. https://www.who.int/data/gho/data/themes/hiv-aids#:~:text=Globally%2C%2037.7%20million%20%5B30.2%E2%80%93,considerably%20between%20countries%20and%20regions.
3. Poynten IM, Grulich AE, Templeton DJ. Sexually transmitted infections in older populations. Curr Opin Infect Dis. 2013;26(1):80–5. https://doi.org/10.1097/QCO.0b013e32835c2173.
4. Levy BR, Ding L, Lakra D, Kosteas J, Niccolai L. Older persons' exclusion from sexually transmitted disease risk-reduction clinical trials. Sex Transm Dis. 2007;34(8):541–4. https://doi.org/10.1097/01.olq.0000253342.75908.05.
5. Chawla N, Sarkar S. Defining "high-risk sexual behavior" in the context of substance use. J Psychosex Health. 2019;1(1):26–31. https://doi.org/10.1177/2631831818822015.
6. Dermen KH, Cooper ML, Agocha VB. Sex-related alcohol expectancies as moderators of the relationship between alcohol use and risky sex in adolescents. J Stud Alcohol. 1998;59(1):71–7. https://doi.org/10.15288/jsa.1998.59.71.
7. McKirnan DJ, Ostrow DG, Hope B. Sex, drugs and escape: a psychological model of HIV-risk sexual behaviours. AIDS Care. 1996;8(6):655–69. https://doi.org/10.1080/09540129650125371.
8. Steele CM, Josephs RA. Alcohol myopia. Its prized and dangerous effects. Am Psychol. 1990;45(8):921–33. https://doi.org/10.1037//0003-066x.45.8.921.
9. Stoner SA, George WH, Peters LM, Norris J. Liquid courage: alcohol fosters risky sexual decision-making in individuals with sexual fears. AIDS Behav. 2007;11(2):227–37. https://doi.org/10.1007/s10461-006-9137-z.
10. Grabovac I, Koyanagi A, Yang L, López-Sánchez GF, McDermott D, Soysal P, Turan Isik A, Veronese N, Smith L. Prospective associations between alcohol use, binge drinking and sexual activity in older adults: the English longitudinal study of ageing. Psychol Sex. 2021;12(3):193–201. https://doi.org/10.1080/19419899.2019.1687581.
11. Schick V, Herbenick D, Reece M, Sanders SA, Dodge B, Middlestadt SE, Fortenberry JD. Sexual behaviors, condom use, and sexual health of Americans over 50: implications for sexual health promotion for older adults. J Sex Med. 2010;7(Suppl 5):315–29. https://doi.org/10.1111/j.1743-6109.2010.02013.x.
12. Lawn W, Aldridge A, Xia R, Winstock AR. Substance-linked sex in heterosexual, homosexual, and bisexual men and women: an online, cross-sectional "global drug survey" report. J Sex Med. 2019;16(5):721–32. https://doi.org/10.1016/j.jsxm.2019.02.018.
13. Blomquist PB, Mohammed H, Mikhail A, Weatherburn P, Reid D, Wayal S, Hughes G, Mercer CH. Characteristics and sexual health service use of MSM engaging in chemsex: results from a large online survey in England. Sex Transm Infect. 2020;96(8):590–5. https://doi.org/10.1136/sextrans-2019-054345.
14. Grabovac I, Meilinger M, Schalk H, Leichsenring B, Dorner TE. Prevalence and associations of illicit drug and polydrug use in people living with HIV in Vienna. Sci Rep. 2018;8(1):8046. https://doi.org/10.1038/s41598-018-26413-5.
15. Jennings A. Knowledge of sexually transmitted infections among older veterans. J Gerontol Geriatr Res. 2015;4(2):1–4. https://doi.org/10.4172/2167-7182.1000203.
16. Lyons A, Heywood W, Fileborn B, Minichiello V, Barrett C, Brown G, Hinchliff S, Malta S, Crameri P. Sexually active older Australian's knowledge of sexually transmitted infections and safer sexual practices. Aust N Z J Public Health. 2017;41(3):259–61. https://doi.org/10.1111/1753-6405.12655.
17. Zablotsky D, Kennedy M. Risk factors and HIV transmission to midlife and older women: knowledge, options, and the initiation of safer sexual practices. J Acquir Immune Defic Syndr. 2003;33;S122–30.

18. Negin J, Martiniuk A, Cumming RG, Naidoo N, Phaswana-Mafuya N, Madurai L, Williams S, Kowal P. Prevalence of HIV and chronic comorbidities among older adults. AIDS (London, England). 2012;26(1):S55–63. https://doi.org/10.1097/QAD.0b013e3283558459.
19. Bergeron CD, Goltz HH, Szucs LE, Reyes JV, Wilson KL, Ory MG, Smith ML. Exploring sexual behaviors and health communication among older women. Health Care Women Int. 2017;38(12):1356–72. https://doi.org/10.1080/07399332.2017.1329308.
20. Lieberman R. HIV in older Americans: an epidemiologic perspective. J Midwifery Womens Health. 2000;45(2):176–82. https://doi.org/10.1016/s1526-9523(00)00002-7.
21. Lindau ST, Schumm LP, Laumann EO, Levinson W, O'Muircheartaigh CA, Waite LJ. A study of sexuality and health among older adults in the United States. N Engl J Med. 2007;357(8):762–74. https://doi.org/10.1056/NEJMoa067423.
22. Rose MA. HIV/AIDS knowledge, perceptions of risk, and behaviors of older adults. Holist Nurs Pract. 1995;10(1):10–7.
23. Pinyopornpanish K, Thanamee S, Jiraporncharoen W, Thaikla K, McDonald J, Aramrattana A, Angkurawaranon C. Sexual health, risky sexual behavior and condom use among adolescents young adults and older adults in Chiang Mai, Thailand: findings from a population based survey. BMC Res Notes. 2017;10(1):682. https://doi.org/10.1186/s13104-017-3055-1.
24. Choe H-S, Lee S-J, Kim CS, Cho Y-H. Prevalence of sexually transmitted infections and the sexual behavior of elderly people presenting to health examination centers in Korea. J Infect Chemother. 2011;17(4):456–61. https://doi.org/10.1007/s10156-010-0191-0.
25. Fish R, Robinson A, Copas A, Jungmann E, Lascar RM. Trends in attendances to genitourinary medicine services by older women. Int J STD AIDS. 2012;23(8):595–6. https://doi.org/10.1258/ijsa.2012.011426.
26. CDC. New HIV infections in the United States [CDC Fact Sheet]. 2012. https://www.cdc.gov/nchhstp/newsroom/docs/2012/HIV-INfections-2007-2010.pdf.
27. Karpiak SE, Lunievicz JL. Age is not a condom: HIV and sexual health for older adults. Curr Sex Health Rep. 2017;9(3):109–15. https://doi.org/10.1007/s11930-017-0119-0.
28. WHO. Sexually transmitted infections (STIs). 2021b. https://www.who.int/news-room/fact-sheets/detail/sexually-transmitted-infections-(stis).
29. Bodley-Tickell AT, Olowokure B, Bhaduri S, White DJ, Ward D, Ross JDC, Smith G, Duggal HV, Goold P. Trends in sexually transmitted infections (other than HIV) in older people: analysis of data from an enhanced surveillance system. Sex Transm Infect. 2008;84(4):312–7. https://doi.org/10.1136/sti.2007.027847.
30. ECDC. Sexually transmitted infections in Europe 1990–2010. Surveillance Report. Surveillance report. Publications Office of the European Union; 2012.
31. ECDC. HIV/AIDS surveillance in Europe 2019: 2018 data. HIV/AIDS surveillance in Europe 2019 [publications Office of the European Union]; WHO Regional Office for Europe; 2019.
32. Mahy M, Autenrieth CS, Stanecki K, Wynd S. Increasing trends in HIV prevalence among people aged 50 years and older: evidence from estimates and survey data. AIDS (London, England). 2014;28(Suppl 4):S453–9. https://doi.org/10.1097/QAD.0000000000000479.
33. Padian NS, Shiboski SC, Glass SO, Vittinghoff E. Heterosexual transmission of human immunodeficiency virus (HIV) in northern California: results from a ten-year study. Am J Epidemiol. 1997;146(4):350–7. https://doi.org/10.1093/oxfordjournals.aje.a009276.
34. Meditz AL, Moreau KL, MaWhinney S, Gozansky WS, Melander K, Kohrt WM, Wierman ME, Connick E. Ccr5 expression is elevated on endocervical CD4+ T cells in healthy postmenopausal women. J Acquir Immune Defic Syndr. 2012;59(3):221–8. https://doi.org/10.1097/QAI.0b013e31823fd215.
35. Lindau ST, Leitsch SA, Lundberg KL, Jerome J. Older women's attitudes, behavior, and communication about sex and HIV: a community-based study. J Womens Health (Larchmt). 2006;15(6):747–53. https://doi.org/10.1089/jwh.2006.15.747.
36. ACRIA. Older adults and sexual health: a guide for aging services providers. 2020. https://www.health.ny.gov/diseases/aids/general/publications/docs/sexual_health_older_adults.pdf.
37. Jacobs RJ, Thomlison B. Self-silencing and age as risk factors for sexually acquired HIV in midlife and older women. J Aging Health. 2009;21(1):102–28. https://doi.org/10.1177/0898264308328646.

38. Pilowsky DJ, Wu L-T. Sexual risk behaviors and HIV risk among Americans aged 50 years or older: a review. Subst Abuse Rehabil. 2015;6:51–60. https://doi.org/10.2147/SAR.S78808.
39. Savasta AM. Hiv: associated transmission risks in older adults—an integrative review of the literature. J Assoc Nurs AIDS Care. 2004;15(1):50–9. https://doi.org/10.1177/1055329003252051.
40. Amin I. Social capital and sexual risk-taking Behaviors among older adults in the United States. J Appl Gerontol. 2016;35(9):982–99. https://doi.org/10.1177/0733464814547048.
41. Tillman JL, Mark HD. HIV and STI testing in older adults: an integrative review. J Clin Nurs. 2015;24(15–16):2074–95. https://doi.org/10.1111/jocn.12797.
42. Chen Z-Q, Zhang G-C, Gong X-D, Lin C, Gao X, Liang G-J, Yue X-L, Chen X-S, Cohen MS. Syphilis in China: results of a national surveillance programme. Lancet (London, England). 2007;369(9556):132–8. https://doi.org/10.1016/S0140-6736(07)60074-9.
43. Haddad N, Robert A, Popovic N, Varsaneux O, Edmunds M, Jonah L, Siu W, Weeks A, Archibald C. Newly diagnosed cases of HIV in those aged 50 years and older and those less than 50: 2008-2017. Can Commun Dis Rep (Releve Des Maladies Transmissibles Au Canada). 2019;45(11):283–8. https://doi.org/10.14745/ccdr.v45i11a02.
44. Saag MS, Gandhi RT, Hoy JF, Landovitz RJ, Thompson MA, Sax PE, Smith DM, Benson CA, Buchbinder SP, Del Rio C, Eron JJ, Fätkenheuer G, Günthard HF, Molina J-M, Jacobsen DM, Volberding PA. Antiretroviral drugs for treatment and prevention of HIV infection in adults: 2020 recommendations of the international antiviral society-USA panel. JAMA. 2020;324(16):1651–69. https://doi.org/10.1001/jama.2020.17025.
45. Giorgi JV, Hultin LE, McKeating JA, Johnson TD, Owens B, Jacobson LP, Shih R, Lewis J, Wiley DJ, Phair JP, Wolinsky SM, Detels R. Shorter survival in advanced human immunodeficiency virus type 1 infection is more closely associated with T lymphocyte activation than with plasma virus burden or virus chemokine coreceptor usage. J Infect Dis. 1999;179(4):859–70. https://doi.org/10.1086/314660.
46. Frazier EL, Sutton MY, Tie Y, Collison M, Do A. Clinical characteristics and outcomes among older women with HIV. J Womens Health (Larchmt). 2018;27(1):6–13. https://doi.org/10.1089/jwh.2017.6380.
47. Silverberg MJ, Leyden W, Horberg MA, DeLorenze GN, Klein D, Quesenberry CP. Older age and the response to and tolerability of antiretroviral therapy. Arch Intern Med. 2007;167(7):684–91. https://doi.org/10.1001/archinte.167.7.684.
48. Balestre E, Eholié SP, Lokossue A, Sow PS, Charurat M, Minga A, Drabo J, Dabis F, Ekouevi DK, Thiébaut R. Effect of age on immunological response in the first year of antiretroviral therapy in HIV-1-infected adults in West Africa. AIDS (London, England). 2012;26(8):951–7. https://doi.org/10.1097/QAD.0b013e3283528ad4.
49. Smith RD, Delpech VC, Brown AE, Rice BD. Hiv transmission and high rates of late diagnoses among adults aged 50 years and over. AIDS (London, England). 2010;24(13):2109–15. https://doi.org/10.1097/QAD.0b013e32833c7b9c.
50. Smith L, Yang L, Veronese N, Soysal P, Stubbs B, Jackson SE. Sexual activity is associated with greater enjoyment of life in older adults. Sex Med. 2019;7(1):11–8. https://doi.org/10.1016/j.esxm.2018.11.001.
51. Bach LE, Mortimer JA, VandeWeerd C, Corvin J. The association of physical and mental health with sexual activity in older adults in a retirement community. J Sex Med. 2013;10(11):2671–8. https://doi.org/10.1111/jsm.12308.
52. Foster V, Clark PC, Holstad MM, Burgess E. Factors associated with risky sexual behaviors in older adults. J Assoc Nurs AIDS Care. 2012;23(6):487–99. https://doi.org/10.1016/j.jana.2011.12.008.
53. Gott M, Hinchliff S. Barriers to seeking treatment for sexual problems in primary care: a qualitative study with older people. Fam Pract. 2003;20(6):690–5. https://doi.org/10.1093/fampra/cmg612.

Lifelong Sexual Practice and Its Influence on Health in Later Life

8

Benny Rana, Lin Yang, and Siniša Grabovac

8.1 Background

8.1.1 Life Expectancy and Aging

Life expectancy has been rapidly increasing across the globe due to various factors such as advances in medicine and medical technology, increases in public health expenditure, socioeconomic development, and increasing understanding of gender and genetics. This has led to individuals living longer, healthier, and productive lives. However, statistics show a dramatic increase in the aging population, with an expectation of two billion individuals being aged 60 years or older by 2050 [1, 2]. According to the World Health Organization (WHO), older adults are defined as individuals over the age of 60 [3]. As stated in the WHO reports on aging and health, between 2015 and 2050, the proportion of the world's population over 60 years will nearly double from 12% to 22% [1].

B. Rana
Department of Cancer Epidemiology and Prevention Research, Cancer Research and Analytics, Cancer Care Alberta, Alberta Health Services, Calgary, AB, Canada

Department of Kinesiology, University of Calgary, Calgary, AB, Canada
e-mail: Benny.Rana@albertahealthservices.ca

L. Yang (✉)
Department of Cancer Epidemiology and Prevention Research, Cancer Research and Analytics, Cancer Care Alberta, Alberta Health Services, Calgary, AB, Canada

Departments of Oncology and Community Health Sciences, University of Calgary, Calgary, AB, Canada
e-mail: Lin.Yang@albertahealthservices.ca

S. Grabovac
Institute for Outcome Research, Centre for Medical Statistics, Informatics and Intelligent Systems, Medical University of Vienna, Vienna, Austria
e-mail: sinisa.s.grabovac@gmail.com

© Springer Nature Switzerland AG 2023
L. Smith, I. Grabovac (eds.), *Sexual Behaviour and Health in Older Adults*, Practical Issues in Geriatrics, https://doi.org/10.1007/978-3-031-21029-7_8

8.1.2 Definition of Sexuality and Its Forms

Sexuality, defined by the WHO and World Association for Sexual Health, is multidimensional and encompasses multiple aspects, including sex, gender identities and roles, sexual orientation, eroticism, pleasure, physical touch, emotional intimacy, close companionship, and reproduction [4, 5]. Sexuality can be experienced and expressed in many ways; for example, through verbal expression including thoughts, fantasies, desires, beliefs, attitudes, values, as well as behaviors, practices, roles, kissing, mutual touching, masturbation, fondling, tenderness, and relationships [6, 7]. Any sexual behavior that is expressed alone or with a partner is influenced by the interaction of biological, psychological, social, economic, political, cultural, legal, historical, religious, and spiritual factors [8]. Emotional and physical sexual pleasure as well as interest in sexual behavior does not diminish with age for most healthy individuals and is rated highly by older adults [9–11]. Even though several studies show that the prevalence of sexual activity decreases with increasing age [12–14], the frequency of other (noncoital) form of sexual expression does not change and to some individuals affection (emotional aspect of sexuality) is more important than sexual intercourse [12, 15].

8.1.3 Myths About Sexuality in Older Adults

Regardless of age, many individuals still have a desire to be close to others, which includes the want and need for intimacy, as well as having an active and satisfying sexual life [16–18]. Unfortunately, there are many different cultural myths, taboos, and preconceived ideas, combined with societal ignorance creating a source of misinformation and stereotypes on sexuality in older individuals [11]. In many countries, older adults are still erroneously considered as asexual individuals who have lost their sexual drive as well as the sexual function [19, 20]. Even though sexual desire and enjoyment change over the lifetime [21, 22], physical and emotional pleasure of sexual intimacy is shown to be significantly related to overall happiness and is an important dimension of successful aging [23, 24]. Several population-based studies have shown that sexuality is an important part of life in many older adults [14, 25, 26].

A systematic review was conducted to examine the attitudes and concerns about sex and sexuality in later life. The review identified three main themes: social legitimacy for sexuality in later life; health, not age, is what truly impacts sexuality; and hegemony of penetrative sex [17]. The themes identified illustrated the complexity and how delicate the relation between aging and sexuality is. The first theme identified describes how older adults have the impression that most people assume they are asexual, leading to them feeling sexually invisible which is based on the idea that society values sexuality in youth and beauty. As individuals age, they internalize these values and norms, leading to feelings of shame, and not wanting to express their sexual needs and desires in the fear of being judged or excluded [17, 27]. The second theme highlighted that health, not age, is what impacts sexuality.

As individuals age, there can be physical limitations or certain health conditions that impact the ability to engage in sexual activity. Furthermore, when approaching healthcare providers to discuss sexual problems, older adults are confronted with stereotypical and narrow views leading to a lack of appropriate counseling and care [17, 27]. The last theme identified in the review is the definition of sexuality for older adults. Due to loss or decrease in sexual function, which leads to feelings of distress, disappointment, frustration, and despair, older adults tend to adopt broader definitions of sexuality and sexual activity [17, 27].

Even though stereotypes regarding sexuality of older adults persist, studies show that older adults regard sexuality as an essential component of life and are engaged in spousal or other intimate relationships [14, 28]. The prevalence of sexual activity may decline with age; however, a substantial number of men and women in their eighth and ninth decade of life still engage in vaginal intercourse, oral sex, and masturbation [14]. Sex and sexuality is an important aspect of life, especially for older adults as it influences their quality of life and the quality of their partnerships [28–30]. Studies indicate that sex in later life is predicted by age and the individuals view towards aging; furthermore, sex in later life has become an indicator of successful aging [31–33]. Overall, there are many different ways to express one's sexuality and to be intimate, even as we age. It is important to address the influence of lifelong sexuality, which encompasses partnership, activity, behavior, attitudes, and function, on health in later life.

8.2 Sexual Practice and Influence on Health

8.2.1 Frequency of Sexual Activities in Older Adults and Its Influence on Health

Sexual practices change over the course of a lifetime, including the changes in frequency of sexual intercourse, the number of sexual partners, and types of sexual activity as well as sexual behavior. Even though there are purported risks associated with sexual activity, studies show that having an active sexual life has been associated with various long-term health benefits [34]. For example, sexual activity and frequent sexual intercourse are positively associated with late-life happiness [7], greater quality of life, and life satisfaction [6, 35, 36]. Moreover, the frequency of sexual intercourse may be just as relevant to global life satisfaction as the subjective quality of the sexual intercourse [37–39]. Both men and women reporting sexual activity in the past years had a significantly higher mean scores of life enjoyment, compared to those who were not sexually active [35]. Furthermore, sexually active men, who had frequent sexual intercourse (greater than two times a month), combined with frequent kissing, petting, or fondling, were associated with greater enjoyment of life [35]. Among sexually active women, frequent kissing, petting, or fondling were also associated with greater enjoyment of life [35]. The frequency of sexual activity varies among seniors around the world. In one study of 1216 older Americans with the mean age of 77.3 years, 30% of the studied participants were sexually active in the past month [40], while in another study from the Netherlands, nearly half of 2374 community-dwelling adults older than 65 years had engaged in sexual activities [41]. Furthermore, in one literature review, some seniors preserved different forms of sexual behavior such as petting, masturbation, caressing, and sexual intercourse in the previous year, where some of them specified participating in everyday sexual practices [37].

8.2.2 Sexual Practice in Older Adults and Its Influence on Health

Scientific research has highlighted many benefits of sexual activity on human health in healthy individuals. Sexual intercourse, as well as foreplay, causes stretching of muscles, hormone fluctuation, and joint movements, which may promote cardiovascular fitness [42, 43]. Moreover, partnered sexual relationship increases bonding (emotional closeness), social integration as well as different psychological and behavioral patterns [44–47]. Participation in sexual activities is also known to reduce stress levels since a cocktail of "happy hormones" (endorphins) is released during the intercourse, while the release of hormone oxytocin (especially while having orgasm) promotes bonding [48].

After sexual intercourse, happy and elevated mood may linger for some time, having a positive impact on human health [49–51]. Such positive body-related feelings of pleasure, happiness, relaxation, and excitement may also facilitate better internal body acceptance/image which inevitably changes as individuals age [52]. For these reasons, sexual activity and frequent sexual intercourse have also been associated with improved mental health, especially in terms of lower levels of depression [53]. The positive implications on mental health can be associated with the perceptions of belonging and intimate support as individuals age [53, 54]. Several studies demonstrated a positive association between sexual activity and increased levels of general cognitive function in older adults [55, 56] as well as satisfaction with their own mental health [54, 57]. Social experiences like sexual activity can have a strong influence on endocrine factors that affect adult neurogenesis; however, further research is needed to explore the role for sexual activity and brain health [54, 58, 59]. Benefits of life-long sexual activity also include heart rate variability, which presents a noninvasive index of the autonomic nervous system and is predictive of first fatal and nonfatal cardiovascular disease [60]. Other benefits of sexual activity include having lower cardiovascular risk [45]. A healthy sex life can overall improve life expectancy where a greater frequency of sexual activity is associated with overall lower mortality [61].

The relationship of sexual practices on health often focuses on adolescents and young adults, not taking into consideration the influence on health for older adults. Several studies showed that sexual activity and sexual well-being in late adulthood is not just important for mental health, relationship satisfaction, and increasing self-confidence, but also proven to help maintain higher energy levels and increase physical activities in older populations [6, 62].

8.2.3 Sexually Transmitted Infections in Older Adults

The Centers for Disease Control and Prevention (CDC) defines sexually transmitted infections (STIs) as infections that are passed from one individual to another through intimate sexual contact [63]. Sexual practices like the number of sexual partners are understudied in the older adult population. The number of sexual partners a person has in their lifetime has been correlated to STIs and other health risks [64]. Even though STIs could occur regardless of age, among older individuals, several STIs such as gonorrhea, syphilis, chlamydia, and HIV have been documented and likely to be underreported [65]. A higher number of lifetime sexual partners has been correlated with sociodemographic and behavioral factors [66]. One study described that the lifetime number of sexual partners is associated with STI acquisition, overall leading to health risks which may affect health in later life [64]. Evidence shows the number of lifetime sexual partners is associated with adverse health outcomes in older adults, where both men and women who had more than ten lifetime number of sexual partners had an increased risk of cancer, coronary heart disease, and stroke [64]. Another study examining the longitudinal analyses of sexual behavior noticed patterns of sexual risk behavior when measuring the number of sexual partners, number of incidents of sexual intercourse, and percentage of condom use. The results of the longitudinal analysis indicate those who have multiple sexual partners over time have an increased risk of having sex without protection against STIs, overall leading to health risks in later life [67].

8.3 Health Issues and Concerns on Sexual Health

Sexual activity and function are closely related to human health, which helps us understand sexuality in later life. In both men and women, normal aging is characterized by physical, physiological, pathological, behavioral, and psychological changes, all of which affect sexual functioning and the ability to have and enjoy sex, especially in older age [14, 45, 68]. Some factors for reduced or stopped sexual activity include age, ill health, loss of job, financial crisis, loss of partner, and loss of family-close friend. In many older adults, aging includes adapting sexual activity to accommodate physical, health, and other life changing situations which can affect libido and sexual capacity [18, 27].

Sexual dissatisfaction and sexual well-being are associated with poor health and may be a warning sign or a consequence of a serious health condition [37, 69–71], such as diabetes, arthritis, urogenital conditions, chronic pain, heart disease, and cancer [72]. Such health conditions can have a negative effect on sexual behavior, resulting in decreased sexual drive, and thus affect an individual's ability to become aroused and have an orgasm. Since sexuality is important for physical and mental health, when left undiagnosed and/or untreated, more problems may occur, such as depression and social isolation [73, 74]. Additionally, chronic illness is known to affect sexual desire as well as function, and the incidence of sexual dysfunction increases with age [14].

In one study of sexuality and health among older adults in the USA, at least half of the sexually active older adults reported at least one sexual problem [14]. In that study, the most prevalent reported sexual problems in women were vaginal lubrication, inability to achieve orgasm, and pain while having sex; while men had problems with achieving and maintaining erection, anxiety about sexual performance, and orgasming disorder (inability to achieve, or achieving orgasm too quickly) [14, 69].

Stigma and the lack of positive attitude towards sexuality in older adults, in addition to being more open to discuss sexual issues, are seen as the biggest barrier for all sexes when approaching healthcare professionals [75–78]. A holistic, confident, and nonjudgmental approach towards sexuality among older age individuals is crucial to empower and openly discuss sex-related issues without shame and fear [75–79].

8.3.1 Health Reasons in Older Women That May Affect Sexual Functioning and Satisfaction

Women's sexual function and satisfaction may be affected by many physiological changes which increase with age. Such changes include and may be related to the endocrine, genitourinary, vascular, and musculoskeletal system [80]. Loss of estrogen, which occurs during menopause, may affect various aspects of women's sexuality causing vaginal dryness, changes in the vaginal bacterial flora, thinning of the labia, shortening of the vagina, and many others [22, 80–82]. Moreover, urogenital vascular changes may affect vaginal lubrication whereas the lack of estrogen production may lead to urogenital atrophy and make sexual penetration painful [80].

8.3.2 Health Reasons in Older Men That May Affect Sexual Functioning and Satisfaction

In the course of aging, men also experience physiological changes which might affect sexual functioning and satisfaction [37]. The most common type of sexual dysfunction in older individuals is erectile dysfunction, with the prevalence ranging from 13.1% to 76.5% across the countries [83–86]. Even though erectile dysfunction is the most frequent cause of sexual dysfunction in older adults, it is not considered to be a normal part of aging and it is frequently a result of various risk factors or illnesses [69, 87]. Decreased levels of testosterones in older men, which is estimated to be 20% in adults between 60 and 69 years old and up to 50% in adults above 80 years of age [88], may lead to erectile dysfunction, decreased sexual desire, slow physical reaction time to sexual arousal as well as more time for completing the sexual activity [80, 89, 90].

8.3.3 Sexual Health Among Older Adults Who Identify as Sexual and Gender Minorities

Sexuality and sexual health are often associated as oppressive relating to shame, myth, judgment, and negativity. Culture and societal influence often categorize sexuality with negativity, describing it through disease, disaster, and dysfunction [31]. Sex negativity is more prevalent in discussions involving marginalized communities. Marginalized communities include sexual and gender minorities, individuals who identify as lesbian, gay, bisexual, asexual, transgender, Two-Spirit, queer, and/or intersex (LGBTQIA2+) [32]. Sexual and gender minorities continue to experience health inequities due to stigma, discrimination, and criminalization, and are understudied and underrepresented in research [33, 34].

Sexual and gender minorities experience inequalities in sexual health, where individual behaviors, structural, socioeconomic, and legal factors play a huge role. Sexual health inequalities among sexual and gender minorities include increased susceptibility to bacterial vaginosis among Lesbian women [35, 36]. Studies also highlighted the prevalence of sexually transmitted infections (STIs) and human immunodeficiency virus (HIV) among sexual and gender minorities [36–41]. Transfeminine and gay and bisexual men have greater vulnerability to sexually transmitted infections and human immunodeficiency virus compared with cisgendered heterosexuals [42, 43]. Furthermore, a study highlighted that transfeminine individuals have an increased risk of human immunodeficiency virus with 49 times greater odds of infection when compared to all adults [44, 45]. This increased risk can be associated with the stigma and discrimination that sexual and gender minorities endure as it can foster unhealthy coping mechanisms including sexual risk behavior, but also leads to decreased access to health care, especially screening and prevention [44].

8.4 Sexual Health and Chronic Conditions Among Older Adults

The burden of chronic diseases has increased due to the increased life expectancy and the growing aging population [91]. This burden has an adverse effect on the overall health of older adults, which may also influence their sexuality. Sexuality and sexual life are often overlooked in older adults. Furthermore, when combined with certain chronic conditions, sexuality may not be addressed and even ignored in society [92].

The prevalent chronic condition, cancer, has shown to have a complex impact on sexuality among older adults [93]. Older adults living with and beyond cancer can experience sexuality-related issues regardless of cancer type or treatment [46–48], significantly impacting sexual motivation, sexual behavior, and sexual pleasure [49,

50]. Unfortunately, sexual health among individuals living with and beyond cancer, regardless of age, is overlooked. Sexual dysfunction is known to be a common side effect of cancer treatment [51–53] and there appears to be a large gender disparity in how physicians discuss sexual health with their patients [54]. Past research shows that individuals living with and beyond cancer experience unmet sexual health needs, which includes lack of communication and information from healthcare providers about sexuality [55, 56, 58]. A current survey conducted on individuals living with and beyond cancer provided insight that suggests providing information regarding sexuality as standard cancer care to enhance communication is needed and wanted by individuals [46]. According to the survey, individuals, especially older adults, want to see practical tips and information about sexuality to meet individual preferences [46]. When considering the growing population of older adults, many barriers are present. Schaller et al. highlighted the barriers for seeking help for sexual issues among older adults and categorized them into five themes: dynamics in communication, understanding of sexuality, knowledge and competence, attitudes, and structural conditions [54].

Older adults, who have been diagnosed with chronic conditions such as cancer, find it difficult to gain information about sexuality through their healthcare providers. Sexual health conversations between healthcare providers and their patients, especially patients who are older in age, need to become normalized within cancer care.

8.5 Conclusion

Sexuality is important for human health and well-being. As the aging population worldwide increases and people live longer and healthier lives, the ability to remain sexually active is a major concern in the lives of many older individuals. There are many forms of sexual behavior and types of sexual activity. When communicating and/or working with older individuals, it is essential not to assume that older individuals are indifferent to intimacy and sexual pleasure, as well as leading a satisfying sexual life. Sexuality and its forms have been known to positively influence physical, emotional, social, and cognitive aspects of human health. Among the older population, sexual dissatisfaction and decreased sexual-related well-being may be a warning sign or consequences of serious health conditions. Sexual health-related problems in older adults are frequent; however, they are scarcely brought to the attention of physicians and other healthcare professionals. Thus, it is important to integrate a safe and nonjudgmental system within healthcare professionals where all sexually active older individuals have access to education, counseling, and treatment on and about sexual risks and safe sexual practices.

References

1. World Health Organization. Ageing and health. 2021. https://www.who.int/news-room/factsheets/detail/ageing-and-health. Accessed 16 Nov 2021.
2. Lima M, Belon A, Barros M. Happy life expectancy among older adults: differences by sex and functional limitations. Rev Saude Publica. 2016;10(26):50.
3. World Health Organization. World report on ageing and health. 2015. https://apps.who.int/iris/handle/10665/186463. Accessed 16 Nov 2021.
4. World Association for Sexual Health. Declaration of sexual rights. 2014. https://worldsexualhealth.net/resources/declaration-of-sexual-rights/. Accessed 16 Nov 2021.
5. World Health Organization. Sexual and reproductive health—defining sexual health. 2006. https://www.who.int/teams/sexual-and-reproductive-health-and-research/key-areas-of-work/sexual-health/defining-sexual-health. Accessed 16 Nov 2021.
6. Skalacka K, Gerymski R. Sexual activity and life satisfaction in older adults. Psychogeriatrics. 2019;19(3):195–201.
7. Blanchflower DG, Oswald AJ. Money, sex and happiness: an empirical study. Scand J Econ. 2004;106(3):393–415.
8. World Health Organization. Sexual health. 2021. https://www.who.int/health-topics/sexual-health#tab=tab_1https://www.cdc.gov/std/default.htm. Accessed 17 Nov 2021.
9. DeLamater J. Sexual expression in later life: a review and synthesis. J Sex Res. 2012;49(2–3):125–41.
10. DeLamater JD, Sill M. Sexual desire in later life. J Sex Res. 2005;42(2):138–49.
11. Foley S. Older adults and sexual health: a review of current literature. Curr Sex Health Rep. 2015;7(2):70–9.
12. Waite LJ, Laumann EO, Das A, et al. Sexuality: measures of partnerships, practices, attitudes, and problems in the National Social Life, health, and aging study. J Gerontol B Psychol Sci Soc Sci. 2009;64(Suppl 1):i56–66.
13. Galinsky AM, McClintock MK, Waite LJ. Sexuality and physical contact in National Social Life, health, and aging project wave 2. J Gerontol B Psychol Sci Soc Sci. 2014;69(Suppl 2):S83–98.
14. Lindau ST, Schumm LP, Laumann EO, et al. A study of sexuality and health among older adults in the United States. N Engl J Med. 2007;357(8):762–74.
15. Muller B, Nienaber CA, Reis O, et al. Sexuality and affection among elderly German men and women in long-term relationships: results of a prospective population-based study. PLoS One. 2014;9(11):e111404.
16. Heidari S. Sexuality and older people: a neglected issue. Reprod Health Matters. 2016;24(48):1–5.
17. Gewirtz-Meydan A, Hafford-Letchfield T, Ayalon L, et al. How do older people discuss their own sexuality? A systematic review of qualitative research studies. Cult Health Sex. 2019;21(3):293–308.
18. National Institute of Aging. Sexuality in later life. 2017. https://www.nia.nih.gov/health/sexuality-later-life. Accessed 17 Nov 2021.
19. Tien-Hyatt JL. Self-perceptions of aging across cultures: myth or reality? Int J Aging Hum Dev. 1986;24(2):129–48.
20. Kalra G, Subramanyam A, Pinto C. Sexuality: desire, activity and intimacy in the elderly. Indian J Psychiatry. 2011;53(4):300–6.
21. Watson WK, Stelle C, Bell N. Older women in new romantic relationships. Int J Aging Hum Dev. 2017;85(1):33–43.

22. Kingsberg SA. The impact of aging on sexual function in women and their partners. Arch Sex Behav. 2002;31(5):431–7.
23. Rowe JW, Kahn RL. Successful aging. Gerontologist. 1997;37(4):433–40.
24. Laumann EO, Paik A, Glasser DB, et al. A cross-national study of subjective sexual well-being among older women and men: findings from the global study of sexual attitudes and behaviors. Arch Sex Behav. 2006;35(2):145–61.
25. Mercer CH, Tanton C, Prah P, et al. Changes in sexual attitudes and lifestyles in Britain through the life course and over time: findings from the National Surveys of sexual attitudes and lifestyles (Natsal). Lancet. 2013;382(9907):1781–94.
26. Mitchell KR, Mercer CH, Ploubidis GB, et al. Sexual function in Britain: Findings from the third National Survey of sexual attitudes and lifestyles (Natsal-3). Lancet. 2013;382(9907):1817–29.
27. Barbara AM, Dobbins M, Brian Haynes R, et al. McMaster optimal aging portal: an evidence-based database for geriatrics-focused health professionals. BMC Res Notes. 2017;10(1):271.
28. Sinković M, Towler L. Sexual aging: a systematic review of qualitative research on the sexuality and sexual health of older adults. Qual Health Res. 2019;29(9):1239–54.
29. Fisher LL, AARP. Sex, romance, and relationships: AARP survey of midlife and older adults. Washington, DC: AARP, Knowledge Management; 2010.
30. Forbes MK, Eaton NR, Krueger RF. Sexual quality of life and aging: a prospective study of a nationally representative sample. J Sex Res. 2017;54(2):137–48.
31. Estill A, Mock SE, Schryer E, et al. The effects of subjective age and aging attitudes on mid- to late-life sexuality. J Sex Res. 2018;55(2):146–51.
32. Štulhofer A, Hinchliff S, Jurin T, et al. Successful aging, change in sexual interest and sexual satisfaction in couples from four European countries. Eur J Ageing. 2019;16(2):155–65.
33. Gewirtz-Meydan A, Hafford-Letchfield T, Benyamini Y, et al. Ageism and sexuality. In: Ayalon L, Tesch-Römer C, editors. Contemporary perspectives on ageism. Cham: Springer International; 2018. p. 149–62.
34. Brody S. The relative health benefits of different sexual activities. J Sex Med. 2010;7(4 Pt 1):1336–61.
35. Smith L, Yang L, Veronese N, et al. Sexual activity is associated with greater enjoyment of life in older adults. Sex Med. 2019;7(1):11–8.
36. Flynn TJ, Gow AJ. Examining associations between sexual behaviours and quality of life in older adults. Age Ageing. 2015;44(5):823–8.
37. DeLamater J, Karraker A. Sexual functioning in older adults. Curr Psychiatry Rep. 2009;11(1):6–11.
38. Lee DM, Vanhoutte B, Nazroo J, et al. Sexual health and positive subjective Well-being in partnered older men and women. J Gerontol B Psychol Sci Soc Sci. 2016;71(4):698–710.
39. Kinsey AC, Pomeroy WR, Martin CE. Sexual behavior in the human male. 1948. Am J Public Health. 2003;93(6):894–8.
40. Matthias RE, Lubben JE, Atchison KA, et al. Sexual activity and satisfaction among very old adults: results from a community-dwelling Medicare population survey. Gerontologist. 1997;37(1):6–14.
41. Freak-Poli R, Kirkman M, De Castro LG, et al. Sexual activity and physical tenderness in older adults: cross-sectional prevalence and associated characteristics. J Sex Med. 2017;14(7):918–27.
42. Frappier J, Toupin I, Levy JJ, et al. Energy expenditure during sexual activity in young healthy couples. PLoS One. 2013;8(10):e79342.
43. Levin RJ. Sexual activity, health and well-being—the beneficial roles of coitus and masturbation. Sex Relatsh Ther. 2007;22(1):135–48.
44. Iveniuk J, O'Muircheartaigh C, Cagney KA. Religious influence on older Americans' sexual lives: a nationally-representative profile. Arch Sex Behav. 2016;45(1):121–31.
45. Liu H, Waite LJ, Shen S, et al. Is sex good for your health? A National Study on partnered sexuality and cardiovascular risk among older men and women. J Health Soc Behav. 2016;57:276–96.

46. Burman B, Margolin G. Analysis of the association between marital relationships and health problems: an interactional perspective. Psychol Bull. 1992;112(1):39–63.
47. Cohen S. Social relationships and health. Am Psychol. 2004;59(8):676–84.
48. Magon N, Kalra S. The orgasmic history of oxytocin: love, lust, and labor. Indian J Endocrinol Metab. 2011;15(Suppl 3):S156–61.
49. Kruger T, Exton MS, Pawlak C, et al. Neuroendocrine and cardiovascular response to sexual arousal and orgasm in men. Psychoneuroendocrinology. 1998;23(4):401–11.
50. Exton MS, Bindert A, Kruger T, et al. Cardiovascular and endocrine alterations after masturbation-induced orgasm in women. Psychosom Med. 1999;61(3):280–9.
51. Kashdan TB, Adams LM, Farmer AS, et al. Sexual healing: daily diary investigation of the benefits of intimate and pleasurable sexual activity in socially anxious adults. Arch Sex Behav. 2014;43(7):1417–29.
52. Jannini EA, Fisher WA, Bitzer J, et al. Is sex just fun? How sexual activity improves health. J Sex Med. 2009;6(10):2640–8.
53. Ganong K, Larson E. Intimacy and belonging: the association between sexual activity and depression among older adults. Soc Mental Health. 2011;1(3):153–72.
54. Brody S, Costa RM. Satisfaction (sexual, life, relationship, and mental health) is associated directly with penile-vaginal intercourse, but inversely with other sexual behavior frequencies. J Sex Med. 2009;6(7):1947–54.
55. Wright H, Jenks RA. Sex on the brain! Associations between sexual activity and cognitive function in older age. Age Ageing. 2016;45(2):313–7.
56. Padoani W, Dello Buono M, Marietta P, et al. Influence of cognitive status on the sexual life of 352 elderly Italians aged 65–105 years. Gerontology. 2000;46(5):258–65.
57. Brody S. Vaginal orgasm is associated with better psychological function. Sex Relatsh Ther. 2007;22(2):173–91.
58. Allen MS. Sexual activity and cognitive decline in older adults. Arch Sex Behav. 2018;47(6):1711–9.
59. Hartmans C, Comijs H, Jonker C. The perception of sexuality in older adults and its relationship with cognitive functioning. Am J Geriatr Psychiatry. 2015;23(3):243–52.
60. Brody S, Preut R. Vaginal intercourse frequency and heart rate variability. J Sex Marital Ther. 2003;29(5):371–80.
61. Cao C, Yang L, Xu T, et al. Trends in sexual activity and associations with all-cause and cause-specific mortality among US adults. J Sex Med. 2020;17(10):1903–13.
62. Smith L, Grabovac I, Yang L, et al. Participation in physical activity is associated with sexual activity in older English adults. Int J Environ Res Public Health. 2019;8:16(3).
63. Centers for Disease Control and Prevention. Sexually transmitted diseases. 2021. https://www.cdc.gov/std/default.htm. Accessed 17 Nov 2021.
64. Grabovac I, Smith L, Yang L, et al. The relationship between chronic diseases and number of sexual partners: an exploratory analysis. BMJ Sex Reprod Health. 2020;46(2):100–7.
65. Johnson BK. Sexually transmitted infections and older adults. J Gerontol Nurs. 2013;39(11):53–60.
66. Jackson SE, Yang L, Veronese N, et al. Sociodemographic and behavioural correlates of lifetime number of sexual partners: findings from the English longitudinal study of ageing. BMJ Sex Reprod Health. 2019;45:138–46.
67. Ashenhurst JR, Wilhite ER, Harden KP, et al. Number of sexual partners and relationship status are associated with unprotected sex across emerging adulthood. Arch Sex Behav. 2017;46(2):419–32.
68. Levine GN, Steinke EE, Bakaeen FG, et al. Sexual activity and cardiovascular disease: a scientific statement from the American Heart Association. Circulation. 2012;125(8):1058–72.
69. Laumann EO, Nicolosi A, Glasser DB, et al. Sexual problems among women and men aged 40-80 y: prevalence and correlates identified in the global study of sexual attitudes and behaviors. Int J Impot Res. 2005;17(1):39–57.
70. Laumann EO, Paik A, Rosen RC. Sexual dysfunction in the United States: prevalence and predictors. JAMA. 1999;281(6):537–44.

71. Camacho ME, Reyes-Ortiz CA. Sexual dysfunction in the elderly: age or disease? Int J Impot Res. 2005;17(Suppl 1):S52–6.
72. Rosen RC, Wing R, Schneider S, et al. Epidemiology of erectile dysfunction: the role of medical comorbidities and lifestyle factors. Urol Clin North Am. 2005;32(4):403–17. v
73. Nicolosi A, Moreira ED Jr, Villa M, et al. A population study of the association between sexual function, sexual satisfaction and depressive symptoms in men. J Affect Disord. 2004;82(2):235–43.
74. Araujo AB, Durante R, Feldman HA, et al. The relationship between depressive symptoms and male erectile dysfunction: cross-sectional results from the Massachusetts male aging study. Psychosom Med. 1998;60(4):458–65.
75. Abramsohn EM, Decker C, Garavalia B, et al. "I'm not just a heart, I'm a whole person here": a qualitative study to improve sexual outcomes in women with myocardial infarction. J Am Heart Assoc. 2013;2(4):e000199.
76. Gott M, Hinchliff S. Barriers to seeking treatment for sexual problems in primary care: a qualitative study with older people. Fam Pract. 2003;20(6):690–5.
77. Hughes AK, Lewinson TD. Facilitating communication about sexual health between aging women and their health care providers. Qual Health Res. 2015;25(4):540–50.
78. Rutte A, Welschen LM, van Splunter MM, et al. Type 2 diabetes patients' needs and preferences for care concerning sexual problems: a cross-sectional survey and qualitative interviews. J Sex Marital Ther. 2016;42(4):324–37.
79. Jobson G. Changing masculinities: land-use, family communication and prospects for working with older men towards gender equality in a livelihoods intervention. Cult Health Sex. 2010;12(3):233–46.
80. Morton L. Sexuality in the older adult. Prim Care. 2017;44(3):429–38.
81. Basson R. The female sexual response: a different model. J Sex Marital Ther. 2000;26(1):51–65.
82. Lund KJ. Menopause and the menopausal transition. Med Clin North Am. 2008;92(5):1253–71. xii
83. Zhang X, Yang B, Li N, et al. Prevalence and risk factors for erectile dysfunction in Chinese adult males. J Sex Med. 2017;14(10):1201–8.
84. Quilter M, Hodges L, von Hurst P, et al. Male sexual function in New Zealand: a population-based cross-sectional survey of the prevalence of erectile dysfunction in men aged 40–70 years. J Sex Med. 2017;14(7):928–36.
85. Oyelade BO, Jemilohun AC, Aderibigbe SA. Prevalence of erectile dysfunction and possible risk factors among men of South-Western Nigeria: a population based study. Pan Afr Med J. 2016;24:124.
86. Ayta IA, McKinlay JB, Krane RJ. The likely worldwide increase in erectile dysfunction between 1995 and 2025 and some possible policy consequences. BJU Int. 1999;84(1):50–6.
87. Freak-Poli R. It's not age that prevents sexual activity later in life. Aust J Ageing. 2020;39(Suppl 1):22–9.
88. Baum NH, Crespi CA. Testosterone replacement in elderly men. Geriatrics. 2007;62(9):15–8.
89. Ni Lochlainn M, Kenny RA. Sexual activity and aging. J Am Med Dir Assoc. 2013;14(8):565–72.
90. Genazzani AR, Gambacciani M, Simoncini T. Menopause and aging, quality of life and sexuality. Climacteric. 2007;10(2):88–96.
91. The Lancet Public Health. Ageing: a 21st century public health challenge? Lancet Public Health. 2017;2(7):e297.
92. Merghati-Khoei E, Pirak A, Yazdkhasti M, et al. Sexuality and elderly with chronic diseases: a review of the existing literature. J Res Med Sci. 2016;21:136.
93. Bates G, Taub RN, West H. Intimacy, body image, and cancer. JAMA Oncol. 2016;2(12):1667.

Medication Use and Sexual Activity in Older Adults

9

Damiano Pizzol, Petre Cristian Ilie, and Nicola Veronese

9.1 Introduction

Medication prescribed for different conditions can affect sexual activity, especially in older adults. The effects can cause sexual dysfunction or can enhance the sexual function [1]. To establish whether medication use is a cause of sexual dysfunction, one needs to find out if the presence of symptoms was prior to medication commencement, if the persistence had a constant duration even after stopping the intake of the medication and if there are other factors that can explain the dysfunction. Such information can be obtained from medical history, physical examination and laboratory tests. It should also be taken into consideration that the dysfunction can sometimes be directly attributable to the diseases for which the patients are being treated, as in the case of depression, which in itself can negatively modify the sexual response [2]. In this chapter we discuss the main drugs affecting sexual activity or prescribed to enhance the sexual function both in older men and women.

D. Pizzol (✉)
Italian Agency for Development Cooperation – Khartum, Khartum, Sudan

P. C. Ilie
Research and Innovation Department, The Queen Elizabeth Hospital Foundation Trust, King's Lynn, UK

N. Veronese
Geriatrics Unit, Department of Internal Medicine and Geriatrics, University of Palermo, Palermo, Italy
e-mail: nicola.veronese@unipa.it

9.2 Men

9.2.1 Medication Affecting Sexual Function

Several types of drugs can have various consequences on sexuality. Men, on whom most of the studies have been conducted, are mainly affected by decreased libido and erectile dysfunction (ED).

One of the main pathophysiologic mechanisms is related to the increase of prolactin hormone [3]. Hyperprolactinaemia would lead to hypogonadism by inhibitory effect on the hypothalamic-pituitary-gonadal axis. The increase in prolactin secretion can be produced by antipsychotics, tricyclic antidepressants, dopamine receptor blockers, some antihypertensives (alfa-methyldopa, Reserpine), oestrogens, opioids, calcium channel blockers (Verapamil) anxiolytics and blockers of H2 histamine receptors [3]. If the antipsychotics cause hyperprolactinaemia by dopamine receptor blockade, serotonin reuptake inhibitors, the most common cause of drug-induced hyperprolactinaemia, do not have a clear mechanism and it seems to be caused by the serotonin indirect effect. Before starting antipsychotics, a baseline prolactin level should be measured. The possible consequences are hypogonadism, gynecomastia, galactorrhoea and low levels of serum testosterone, as well as a decrease in libido, infertility and decrease in the sperm volume and quality (oligospermia) [4]. The loss of libido can be caused by a multitude of drugs, including barbiturates, benzodiazepines, lithium, neuroleptics, tricyclic antidepressants, monoamine oxidase inhibitors, lipid lowering agents, serotonin reuptake inhibitors, anticholinergics, antihistamines, progesterone and oestrogen, anorectic agents as fenfluramine and diethylpropion, glucocorticoids and antifungal ketoconazole [5, 6]. Among the antihypertensives, two diuretics have the greatest effects on sexual desire: chlorothiazide, which induces mainly impotence due to its vasodilating action and the alteration of blood pressure in the penis, and spironolactone, which causes a decrease of libido, impotence and gynecomastia [7]. Interestingly, also clonidine, an α2-adrenergic receptor agonist, can cause a decrease in desire, but it seems that this is more a consequence of the difficulties in erection and ejaculation, which are the main effects of the substance [8]. Even further, some antihistamine drugs may also decrease libido due to their sedative effect and can also cause ED due to their further action on autonomic nervous system receptors [9].

Antidepressant drugs have real inhibitory effects on sexuality and, in particular, tricyclic derivatives raise prolactin rates while lithium carbonate causes a decrease of sexual desire. Furthermore, MAOIs and "second generation" antidepressants also have negative effects on sexuality, which, however, generally tend to diminish or disappear after the first weeks of treatment [6]. Anti-epileptics can lead to a drop in libido, but it is not clear whether this is a direct effect of the drugs [10]. The adrenergic receptor blockers, which are used as antihypertensives, for some particular heart ailments and for asthma, affect the male sexual response, both with ED and ejaculation disorders [11]. In particular, prazosin can cause impotence and rare cases of priapism [11]. Priapism, a persistent and often painful erection not accompanied by sexual desire, can also be caused by other drugs, such as chlorpromazine, thiothixene, fluphenazine, clozapine, and thioridazine [12]. Thioridazine, clomipramine and imipramine can also cause painful orgasms [12].

Antipsychotic drugs, due to their antiadrenergic and/or anticholinergic and antidopaminergic effects, can induce both decreases in desire and inhibition of erection and ejaculation: some phenothiazines affect the latter, while thioxanthenes and, in particular, benzamides increase prolactin rates, decreasing libido [13].

ED may also be due to: (a) antihypertensive drugs such as digoxin, which lowers testosterone levels and elevates those of oestrogen causing gynecomastia; (b) metronidazole antibiotic; (c) histamine H2 receptors blockers; (d) natural alkaloids (atropine); (e) other anticholinergics such as bantine, probantine and compounds ammonia; and (f) steroidal anti-inflammatories, which, if used for prolonged treatments together with cortisone derivatives, can cause a libido decrease [14, 15].

Finally, ED may also be determined by barbiturates, benzodiazepines, tricyclic antidepressants, and endocrine drugs, such as progestins, when used in the treatment of benign prostatic hyperplasia, and anti-androgens [15].

9.2.2 Enhancing Sexual Activity

Advanced age often leads to a condition called late-onset hypogonadism (LOH) characterised by low levels of testosterone (T) in men [16]. Low level of T may cause many symptoms including fatigue, loss of energy, depressed mood, decreased libido and ED [17]. Thus, T replacement therapy is able to significantly mitigate these symptoms. Moreover, T treatment may also augment the benefits of lifestyle interventions: T treatment of middle-aged obese men with low T level subjected to a weight loss programme prevented the diet-associated loss of lean mass, while maintaining the loss of body fat [18]. Furthermore, T therapy is associated with multiple benefits highly relevant to the patient including amelioration of sexual function, depressive mood, muscle function, anaemia, vertebral and femoral bone mineral density (BMD), and body composition [19]. Different formulations of T are available, including oral, buccal, nasal, subdermal, transdermal and intramuscular, for replacement therapy to relieve symptoms and signs of androgen deficiency in men with LOH [20].

ED is considered an age-related disease, affecting 20% of men aged >40 years and with prevalence across age groups as follows: 20% before age 30, 25% at age 30–39, 40% at age 40–49, 60% at age 50–59, 80% at age 60–69, and 90% at age 70 or more [21]. Various first-line treatment options are available, including lifestyle modification, testosterone supplementation, psychosexual and couple therapy, phosphodiesterase type 5 inhibitors (PDE5Is), vacuum erection devices and topical or intra-urethral agents (alprostadil) [22]. Lifestyle modification looks at addressing the modifiable risk factors associated with ED: lack of exercise, smoking, diabetes mellitus, dyslipidaemia, obesity and metabolic syndrome. More better quality studies are required to prove the value of this approach. Recent evidence showed that all PDE5Is were superior, when compared to placebo, in treating ED and that lower dosages had comparable effects to higher dosages [22]. Different PDE5Is seem to have comparable efficacy but they appeared more efficacious when used in combination with alpha blockers or psychological interventions [23]. Despite their high effectiveness, many issues should be considered before their administration including etiologic considerations, performance status, safety, adverse effects, bad experiences with previous treatment, cost and satisfaction [24]. The most common adverse effects of PDE5i are headache, flushing, dyspepsia and upper respiratory tract symptoms [25]. Moreover, especially some clinical conditions should be taken into account before administration. First of all, from a cardiological point of view there are clear cautions and contraindications for PDE5Is in patients with unstable angina, severe congestive heart failure, or uncontrolled hypertension, those at high risk for arrhythmias, and those receiving nitrates or any other form of nitric oxide donors [25]. In addition, PDE5Is undergo extensive tubular reabsorption in the kidney, thus leading to minimal renal clearance and excretion. Thus, in men with chronic renal insufficiency (creatinine clearance <30 mL/min), it is recommended to initiate PDE5I therapy at a lower dose and titrate up as tolerated because of decreased drug clearance [25]. Finally, PDE5Is undergo rapid metabolism and excretion in the liver primarily through the CYP3A, CYP2C9, CYP2C19 and CYP2D6 pathways. Considering that mild and moderate hepatic impairments significantly decrease oral clearance and increase maximum concentration, it is recommended to initiate therapy at lower doses and titrating up as tolerated [25].

Vacuum erection devices might have an efficacy in achieving an erection of 90%, but satisfaction rates are between 27% and 94% and they could be associated with tissue damages [26]. Prostaglandins intracavernous injections can be an option for patients not responding to previously described treatment options. The success rate for achieving an erection can be as high as 85% and, considering the topical action, there are few side effects [26].

9.3 Women

9.3.1 Medication Affecting Sexual Function

As described above for men, the increase in prolactin secretion may affect the sexual health also in women. In fact, it can cause amenorrhea and galactorrhoea, with a decrease of libido and it can be produced by tricyclic antidepressants, by some anxiolytics and by drugs blocking the histamine H2 receptors [27, 28]. As reported for men, antidepressant drugs affect sexual activity deeply and, in particular, tricyclic derivatives raise prolactin rates while lithium carbonate causes decrease of sexual desire [29, 30]. Furthermore, as for men, MAOIs and "second generation" antidepressants also have negative effects on sexuality, which, however, generally tend to diminish or disappear after the first weeks of treatment [6]. Anti-epileptics can lead to a drop in libido, but it is not clear whether this is a direct effect of the drugs [10].

In some cases a decreased libido and vaginal dryness have been reported in women taking oral contraceptives: the pill produces a reduction in androgen levels, but these symptoms are not experienced by all women and, therefore, the data cannot be completely generalised [31].

Finally, steroidal anti-inflammatories, especially if used for prolonged treatments together with cortisone derivatives, can cause a libido decrease as described also for men [14, 15, 32].

9.3.2 Medication Enhancing Sexual Activity

Oestrogen treatment in women has been shown to lead to increased frequency of sexual activity and improved sexual interest and arousal. Moreover, they can help also in terms of vaginal dryness or pain during intercourse [33]. Long-term safety, optimal types, doses and routes of therapy, however, remain unclear [34]. Considering that hormone replacement therapy is not without potential risks such as the increased probability of breast cancer and stroke, currently, it is only recommended for short-term use [35].

In addition to these treatments, acute exercise as exercise manipulation improves physical sexual arousal in women taking antidepressants by increasing sympathetic nervous system activity and vaginal sexual arousal [36].

9.4 Conclusions

A wide range of drug categories are well known in affecting sexual activity both in women and men as summarised in Table 9.1. In contrast, efficacious active ingredients are studied and utilised in order to improve the sexual life and, thus, the quality of life especially in older people. In addition to the medicaments reviewed in this chapter, alcohol and nicotine are two widespread substances to consider regarding sexual health. On one side, alcohol, which in small quantities increases desire and decreases inhibitions, when taken for a prolonged period of time and in high doses, can decrease libido, causing ED, poor lubrication, arousal dysfunction and orgasm inhibition. Nicotine, maybe due to its vasoconstricting effects, can induce ED.

To date, studies have focused more on the effects of different substances on men, although many drugs affect the performance and sexual behaviour of both sexes depending on the type of drug, the amount consumed, the length of the period of use, environmental factors and individual expectations.

Regardless of the availability of safe and effective drugs, the first-line treatment of sexual dysfunction should remove the causing conditions such as treating obesity, type 2 diabetes (T2DM) or metabolic syndrome and the promotion of healthy lifestyle and diet.

Table 9.1 Main drugs affecting sexual functioning

Drug category	Active ingredient	Possible effects of active ingredient	Possible effects of drug category
Antihypertensives	Spironolactone digoxin	Gynecomastia	Libido decrease
	Clonidine methyldopa	Erectile dysfunction, gynecomastia in men Orgasm delay or absence in women	Erectile dysfunction
	Reserpine hydralazine Hydrochlorothiazide Chlorothiazide		
Adrenergic receptor blockers (Alpha-blockers) (Beta-blockers)	Phenoxybenzamine Prazosin Propranolol	Dry ejaculation Priapism	Libido decrease Erectile dysfunction
Antidepressants (SSRI) (Tricyclics) (MAOIs) ("Second generation")	Sertraline paroxetine Fluoxetine	Spontaneous erections, priapism, penile and vaginal anaesthesia	Libido decrease Erectile dysfunction Orgasmic difficulties
	Amitriptyline, doxepin Isocarboxazid, Phenelzine, tranylcypromine		
	Trazodone	Priapism (including clitoral), spontaneous erections	
Antipsychotics (Phenothiazines) (Thioxanthenes) (Benzamides) (Butyrophenones)	Thioridazine, chlorpromazine	Inhibition of erection and ejaculation, priapism	Libido decrease Orgasmic difficulties
	Chlorprothixene, Sulpiride, Levosulpiride, Sultopride, Tiapride haloperidol	Amenorrhea and galactorrhoea in women; gynecomastia and erectile deficits in men	
Anxiolytics (Benzodiazepines)	Clonazepam, diazepam, Flurazepam, lorazepam, Chlordiazepoxide		Libido decrease Erectile dysfunction Orgasm delay or absence

Legend: *MAOIs* monoamine oxidase inhibitors, *SSRI* selective serotonin reuptake inhibitor

References

1. Lindau ST, Schumm LP, Laumann EO, Levinson W, O'Muircheartaigh CA, Waite LJ. A study of sexuality and health among older adults in the United States. N Engl J Med. 2007;357(8):762–74.
2. Yaqoob S, Yaseen M, Abdullah H, Jarullah FA, Khawaja UA. Sexual dysfunction and associated anxiety and depression in female hemodialysis patients: a cross-sectional study at Karachi Institute of Kidney Diseases. Cureus. 2020;12(8):e10148.

3. Kennedy SH, Rizvi S. Sexual dysfunction, depression, and the impact of antidepressants. J Clin Psychopharmacol. 2009;29(2):157–64.
4. Werneke U, Northey S, Bhugra D. Antidepressants and sexual dysfunction. Acta Psychiatr Scand. 2006;114(6):384–97.
5. Sanchez C, Hyttel J. Comparison of the effects of antidepressants and their metabolites on reuptake of biogenic amines and on receptor binding. Cell Mol Neurobiol. 1999;19:467–89.
6. Yamada M, Yasuhara H. Clinical pharmacology of MAO inhibitors: safety and future. Neurotoxicology. 2004;25:215–21.
7. Morrissette DL, Skinner MH, Hoffman BB, et al. Effects of antihypertensive drugs atenolol and nifedipine on sexual function in older men: A placebo-controlled, crossover study. Arch Sex Behav. 1993;22:99–109.
8. Calabro RS, Bramanti P. Intrathecal clonidine administration and erectile dysfunction: what is the link? Pain Physician. 2013;16(2):E119–20.
9. Hosseinzadeh Zoroufchi B, Doustmohammadi H, Mokhtari T, Abdollahpour A. Benzodiazepines related sexual dysfunctions: A critical review on pharmacology and mechanism of action. Rev Int Androl. 2021;19(1):62–8.
10. Najafi MR, Ansari B, Zare M, Fatehi F, Sonbolestan A. Effects of antiepileptic drugs on sexual function and reproductive hormones of male epileptic patients. Iran J Neurol. 2012;11(2):37–41.
11. Scharf MB, Mayleben DW. Comparative effects of prazosin and hydrochlorothiazide on sexual function in hypertensive men. Am J Med. 1989;86(1B):110–2.
12. Hsu JH, Shen WW. Male sexual side effects associated with antidepressants: a descriptive clinical study of 32 patients. Int J Psychiatry Med. 1995;25(2):191–201.
13. Montejo AL, Montejo L, Navarro-Cremades F. Sexual side-effects of antidepressant and antipsychotic drugs. Curr Opin Psychiatry. 2015;28(6):418–23.
14. Drobnis EZ, Nangia AK. Cardiovascular/pulmonary medications and male reproduction. Adv Exp Med Biol. 2017;1034:103–30.
15. Ricci E, Parazzini F, Mirone V, Imbimbo C, Palmieri A, Bortolotti A, Di Cintio E, Landoni M, Lavezzari M. Current drug use as risk factor for erectile dysfunction: results from an Italian epidemiological study. Int J Impot Res. 2003;15(3):221–4.
16. Braga PC, Pereira SC, Ribeiro JC, Sousa M, Monteiro MP, Oliveira PF, Alves MG. Late-onset hypogonadism and lifestyle-related metabolic disorders. Andrology. 2020;8:1530.
17. Hijazi RA, Cunningham GR. Andropause: is androgen replacement therapy indicated for the aging male? Annu Rev Med. 2005;56:117–37.
18. Bhasin S, Brito JP, Cunningham GR, et al. Testosterone therapy in men with hypogonadism: an endocrine society clinical practice guideline. J Clin Endocrinol Metab. 2018;103(5):1715–44.
19. Grossmann M, Matsumoto AM. A perspective on middle-aged and older men with functional hypogonadism: focus on holistic management. J Clin Endocrinol Metab. 2017;102(3):1067–75.
20. Barbonetti A, D'Andrea S, Francavilla S. Testosterone replacement therapy. Andrology. 2020;8(6):1551–66. https://doi.org/10.1111/andr.12774.
21. Cheng JYW, Ng EML, Chen RYL, et al. Prevalence of erectile dysfunction in Asian populations: a meta-analysis. Int J Impot Res. 2007;19:229–44.
22. Chen L, Staubli SEL, Schneider MP, et al. Phosphodiesterase 5 inhibitors for the treatment of erectile dysfunction: a trade-off network meta-analysis. Eur Urol. 2015;68:674–80.
23. Choi H, Kim HJ, Bae JH, et al. A meta-analysis of long-versus short-acting phosphodiesterase 5 inhibitors: comparing combination use with a-blockers and a-blocker monotherapy for lower urinary tract symptoms and erectile dysfunction. Int Neurourol J. 2015;19:237–45.
24. Bakr AM, El-Sakka AA, El-Sakka AI. Considerations for prescribing pharmacotherapy for the treatment of erectile dysfunction. Expert Opin Pharmacother. 2021;22:821–34.
25. Yafi FA, Sharlip ID, Becher EF. Update on the safety of phosphodiesterase type 5 inhibitors for the treatment of erectile dysfunction. Sex Med Rev. 2018;6(2):242–52.
26. European Association of Urology. Male sexual dysfunction. https://uroweb.org/guideline/male-sexual-dysfunction/#3. Accessed Jan 2021.

27. Chen LW, Chen MY, Lian ZP, Lin HS, Chien CC, Yin HL, Chu YH, Chen KY. Amitriptyline and sexual function: A systematic review updated for sexual health practice. Am J Mens Health. 2018;12(2):370–9.
28. Pontiroli AE, De Castro e Silva E, Mazzoleni F, Alberetto M, Baio G, Pellicciotta G, De Pasqua A, Stella L, Girardi AM, Pozza G. The effect of histamine and H1 and H2 receptors on prolactin and luteinizing hormone release in humans: sex differences and the role of stress. J Clin Endocrinol Metab. 1981;52(5):924–8.
29. Ghadirian AM, Annable L, Bélanger MC. Lithium, benzodiazepines, and sexual function in bipolar patients. Am J Psychiatry. 1992;149(6):801–5.
30. Montejo-González AL, Llorca G, Izquierdo JA, Ledesma A, Bousoño M, Calcedo A, Carrasco JL, Ciudad J, Daniel E, De la Gandara J, Derecho J, Franco M, Gomez MJ, Macias JA, Martin T, Perez V, Sanchez JM, Sanchez S, Vicens E. SSRI-induced sexual dysfunction: fluoxetine, paroxetine, sertraline, and fluvoxamine in a prospective, multicenter, and descriptive clinical study of 344 patients. J Sex Marital Ther. 1997;23(3):176–94.
31. de Castro Coelho F, Barros C. The potential of hormonal contraception to influence female sexuality. Int J Reprod Med. 2019;2019:9701384.
32. Genazzani A. Sex steroids impact on female sexuality: peripheral and central effects. Theol Sex. 2008;17suppl1:S18.
33. Potter N, Panay N. Vaginal lubricants and moisturizers: a review into use, efficacy, and safety. Climacteric. 2020;24:19–24.
34. Dennerstein L, Alexander JL, Kotz K. The menopause and sexual functioning: a review of the population-based studies. Annu Rev Sex Res. 2003;14:64–82.
35. Warren MP, Halpert S. Hormone replacement therapy: controversies, pros and cons. Best Pract Res Clin Endocrinol Metab. 2004;18:317–32.
36. Lorenz TA, Meston CM. Acute exercise improves physical sexual arousal in women taking antidepressants. Ann Behav Med. 2012;43(3):352–61.

Barriers to Sexual Activity in Older Adults

10

Nicola Veronese and Damiano Pizzol

10.1 Introduction

In a seminal paper, Langer proposes that all people are sexual beings, and that sexuality continues through the lifespan, even if expressions and attitudes of sexuality change over time [1]. In several industrialized countries, it is known that older people are living longer and longer [2]. Furthermore, many older people report greater feelings of solitude and loneliness [3]. It was reported that privacy, considering that families are smaller than previously and adult children are less likely to cohabit, permits older people to express their feelings for each other [4]. However, in modern culture, where youth and sexual activity are synonymous with a good quality of life, the sexual activity of older people is under-researched, under-discussed, and poorly understood and several barriers are present for sexual activity in older persons [5].

In this chapter, we will report and describe the most important barriers to sexual activity in older adults, considering some suggestions to overcome them.

10.2 Barriers to Sexual Activity in Older People

10.2.1 Lack of Positive Social Policy

The topic of sexual activity is of relevance in the world. For this reason the World Health Organization (WHO), one of the most authoritative organisations in health

N. Veronese (✉)
Geriatrics Unit, Department of Internal Medicine and Geriatrics, University of Palermo, Palermo, Italy
e-mail: nicola.veronese@unipa.it

D. Pizzol
Italian Agency for Development Cooperation – Khartum, Khartum, Sudan

care, produced two reports on sexual activity: *Measuring Sexual Health* and *A Framework for Action* [6, 7]. Unfortunately, neither investigates or reports anything on sexual activity in older people [5]. In this sense, only some bulletins of the WHO were proposed for older people [8]. A similar statement can be proposed in national settings. Given this background, our suggestion is to practically develop some guidelines/indications for sexual activity, specific for older people with an international resonance and, then, to implement these indications in national settings.

10.2.2 Partner Availability

Partner availability is an important topic among the possible barriers to sexual activity in older persons, particularly in the case of women over 75 years who are single, divorced, or widowed [4]. This figure is counterbalanced by an increased availability of partners for single older heterosexual men, due to the differences in life expectancy between the genders [5]. The lack of partner availability is probably the greatest barrier to sexual activity in older people [9]. It is reported that the loss of a partner or lack of partner during advanced age has a relevant effect on an individual's desire to engage in sexual intimacy. For example, in a study of 44 older participants, the authors found that people who felt sex had no importance to them did not have partners and, additionally, felt they would not have another partner [10]. The issue of availability of a partner in advanced age does have a relevant effect on older people, since sexual deprivation reduces quality of life, but choosing to become celibate is likely to cause less unhappiness than enforced celibacy [11].

The best intervention for overcoming the problem of lack of a partner is, probably, to increase the possibility of social interactions among older people. It is, in fact, reported that older people have a greater need compared to younger subjects of tenderness and care and eroticism, while sexual intercourse itself is less important and, therefore, the possibility to increase social moments is of importance [12].

In our opinion, some words should be spent for sexual minority older people that, as expected, have significantly more barriers (such as discrimination) to sexual expression [13, 14]. Sexual activities in this population for gay men, most commonly include oral sex and kissing, as for lesbian women, mutual masturbation, oral sex, and vaginal penetration with fingers are most common [15].

10.2.3 Psychological Factors

After the lack of a partner, psychological factors are probably the most important barriers to sexual activity in older people. Interestingly, a survey made about 20 years ago reported that a consistent part of older people think that sex is less important as they age, but they did not agree that sex is only for younger people [16].

In older people who had liberal and positive attitudes, a sense of self-worth, and psychological well-being there was a greater interest in sexual activity and in sexual satisfaction [15, 17].

Desire is frequently mentioned in the studies present in the literature. Unfortunately, there is little clarity in definition, but older women are less likely to report sexual desire and there is a positive relationship between desire and engaging in sexual behavior [4]. This feeling is supported by other studies finding that a reduction in sexual interest and desire is associated with aging, being reported more frequently in women than men [5, 18]. The reasons for this is unclear, but probably current stress, life changes, and previous negative experience may influence sexual desire and satisfaction [9].

In Western culture, it is widely thought that sex is only for the young [19]. The specter of the stereotypical "dirty old man" and "frigid older woman" unfortunately remains with this type of ageism being a form of societal prejudice as it is not based on biological facts of aging [5]. These beliefs remain, despite a better understanding of sexuality and effective treatment for sexual dysfunctions [11].

In an important work, Weeks et al. suggest that society's normative evaluation of the retained capacity for sex, despite older age, is a relevant determinant in sexual activity [11]. It is likely that ageism, an increasing sensation in modern societies, has an impact on what is taboo and its restrictions also focus on what people should not imagine, resulting in some negative feelings, making sexual activity less enjoyable for older persons [20].

Given this background, it appears important to overcome psychological barriers to sexual activity in older subjects. A first attempt could be to discuss with a prepared person this aspect, e.g., with a psychologist. Some research, in fact, has reported that this intervention can improve sexual satisfaction, particularly reducing the shame and the possible barriers to sexual activity in older people [21]. A second option could be to fight against ageism, a relevant problem in current geriatric medicine that often leads to wrong ideas and perceptions in society [22].

10.2.4 Difficulties Interacting with Health Professionals

It is recognized that sexuality and sexual health needs are under-assessed in general healthcare practice as well as geriatric medicine [10]. One study reported that nurses are often the first health professionals that older people talk to and the attitude of the nurse may affect the outcomes of a consultation [23]. For example, some difficulties may occur if the patient has known the health professional for a number of years [23]. Other research reports that nurses' discomfort with the subject may cause them to unconsciously limit interactions that would promote a discussion of the person's sexual needs [24]. Some health professionals should acknowledge their difficulties about discussing sexuality, particularly in older people, and realize that we are all influenced by societal and cultural messages about sexuality [9].

Some other authors reported that we are not raising the issue of sexual needs with older adults suggesting that issues of sexuality have been included as specialist clinical interventions or obscure research topics [10]. Of importance, even when a specialist is consulted, much of the sex therapy literature tends to focus on depersonalized and goal-orientated models of sexuality, which may not be appropriate for older people [25]. Moreover, talking to older people about sex is a challenge for many health professionals, indicating that discussions should be undertaken when the person is fully clothed using softly phrased open-ended questions [18, 26].

There is evidence that older people are less likely to use condoms [10] and that the prevalence of sexually transmitted diseases is increasing in later life further indicating that the need for education on safer sex is needed across all ages [27].

Moreover, health professionals should know that older patients may use terminology in imprecise ways. Besides, confidentiality is a crucial issue in order to establish a trusting doctor-patient relationship and to include sexuality as a basic aspect of health [10]. In this regard, health professionals are required to have an understanding about the evidence base to support sexual activity [5].

Several strategies are proposed by the literature for better discussing with older patients regarding sexuality. For example, Zeiss and Kasl-Godley report that health professionals should use information sensitively to guide discussions about sexuality [17]. Similarly, Peate reports that attitudes to sexual health can play an influential and significant role in older people's sexual identity [23]. While a good medical history is of importance, discussions on sexual activities and sexuality should be less about the details and more about the beliefs/ideas related to sexual activity, encouraging a large definition of and considering a range of sexual behaviors and not concentrating only on sexual intercourse [5]. However, it is important to remember that experiencing sexual dysfunction, is not part of healthy aging, but a complex set of medical conditions (including medications), that is further impacted by culture, expectations, definition of problems, and recognition by healthcare providers [5].

The difficulty to discuss sex in older age is, finally, dramatical in nursing homes or other similar long term care facilities. Sexuality is overall increasing among nursing home residents, but several factors preclude its discussion with healthcare professionals including stigma and presence of cognitive impairment [28, 29].

10.2.5 Physical Conditions

Physical weaknesses and disability both in terms of pain in different parts of the body and neurological disorders and diseases could represent major obstacles to sexual desire [30]. Moreover, older women may verify a decline in sexuality due to menopause and vaginal dryness that represent a natural phenomenon that impede sexuality in aging women. On the other side, the loss of libido and/or sexual potency in males is a major concern that can undermine men's quality of life. It is particularly frustrating when, in presence of libido, erectile dysfunction does not allow sexual satisfaction. The best-case scenario for a couple is the achievement of menopause and andropause at the same time to avoid a couple imbalance but it rarely occurs. Also, for this, improvements in terms of social and health assistance with adequate professionals are needed.

10.3 Conclusions

Barriers to sexual activity in older people are several, including lack of positive social policy, partner availability, and psychological factors. Healthcare professionals have a pivotal role in discussing barriers to sexual activity in older adults and, in this sense, more knowledge and education should be undertaken by those assisting older people.

References

1. Langer N. Late life love and intimacy. Educ Gerontol. 2009;35(8):752–64.
2. Jeune B. Living longer—but better? Aging Clin Exp Res. 2002;14(2):72–93.
3. Solmi M, Veronese N, Galvano D, Favaro A, Ostinelli EG, Noventa V, et al. Factors associated with loneliness: an umbrella review of observational studies. J Affect Disord. 2020;271:131.
4. DeLamater J, Hyde JS, Fong M-C. Sexual satisfaction in the seventh decade of life. J Sex Marital Ther. 2008;34(5):439–54.
5. Garrett D. Psychosocial barriers to sexual intimacy for older people. Br J Nurs. 2014;23(6):327–31.
6. World Health Organization. Framework for action on interprofessional education and collaborative practice. World Health Organization; 2010.
7. World Health Organization. Measuring sexual health: conceptual and practical considerations and related indicators. World Health Organization; 2010.
8. Lusti-Narasimhan M, Beard JR. Sexual health in older women. Bull World Health Organ. 2013;91:707–9.
9. Skultety K. Addressing issues of sexuality with older couples. Generations. 2007;31(3):31–7.
10. Gott M, Hinchliff S. How important is sex in later life? The views of older people. Soc Sci Med. 2003;56(8):1617–28.
11. Weeks DJ. Sex for the mature adult: health, self-esteem and countering ageist stereotypes. Sex Relatsh Ther. 2002;17(3):231–40.
12. von Humboldt S, Ribeiro-Gonçalves JA, Costa A, Low G, Leal I. Sexual expression in old age: how older adults from different cultures express sexually? Sexuality research and social. Policy. 2020;
13. Schwartz P, Diefendorf S, McGlynn-Wright A. Sexuality in aging. In: APA handbook of sexuality and psychology. Vol. 1: Person-based approaches. American Psychological Association; 2014. p. 523–551.
14. Jackson SE, Hackett RA, Grabovac I, Smith L, Steptoe A. Perceived discrimination, health and wellbeing among middle-aged and older lesbian, gay and bisexual people: a prospective study. PLoS One. 2019;14(5):e0216497.
15. Grabovac I, Smith L, McDermott DT, Stefanac S, Yang L, Veronese N, et al. Well-being among older gay and bisexual men and women in England: a cross-sectional population study. J Am Med Dir Assoc. 2019;20(9):1080–5. e1
16. AARP. AARP/modern maturity sexuality study. Washington, DC: AARP; 1999.
17. Zeiss A, Kasl-Godley J. Sexuality in older adults' relationships. Generations. 2001;25(2):18–25.

18. Pariser SF, Niedermier JA. Sex and the mature woman. J Women's Health. 1998;7(7):849–59.
19. Cooper ML, Shapiro CM, Powers AM. Motivations for sex and risky sexual behavior among adolescents and young adults: a functional perspective. J Pers Soc Psychol. 1998;75(6):1528.
20. Gewirtz-Meydan A, Hafford-Letchfield T, Benyamini Y, Phelan A, Jackson J, Ayalon L. Ageism and sexuality. Contemporary perspectives on ageism. Cham: Springer; 2018. p. 149–62.
21. Dhingra I, De Sousa A, Sonavane S. Sexuality in older adults: clinical and psychosocial dilemmas. Journal of Geriatric Mental Health. 2016;3(2):131.
22. Wyman MF, Shiovitz-Ezra S, Bengel J. Ageism in the health care system: providers, patients, and systems. Contemporary perspectives on ageism. Cham: Springer; 2018. p. 193–212.
23. Peate I. Sexuality and sexual health promotion for the older person. Br J Nurs. 2004;13(4):188–93.
24. Mueller IW. Common questions about sex and sexuality in elders. Am J Nurs. 1997;97(7):61–4.
25. Armstrong LL. Barriers to intimate sexuality: concerns and meaning-based therapy approaches. Humanist Psychol. 2006;34(3):281–98.
26. Bauer M, Haesler E, Fetherstonhaugh D. Let's talk about sex: older people's views on the recognition of sexuality and sexual health in the health-care setting. Health Expect. 2016;19(6):1237–50.
27. Xu F, Schillinger JA, Aubin MR, Louis MES, Markowitz LE. Sexually transmitted diseases of older persons in Washington state. Sex Transm Dis. 2001;28(5):287–91.
28. Doll GM. Sexuality in nursing homes: practice and policy. J Gerontol Nurs. 2013;39(7):30–7.
29. Smith L, Grabovac I, Yang L, López-Sánchez GF, Firth J, Pizzol D, et al. Sexual activity and cognitive decline in older age: a prospective cohort study. Aging Clin Exp Res. 2020;32(1):85–91.
30. Gharibi T, Gharibi T, Ravanipour M. Facilitators and barriers affecting sexual desire in elderly Iranian women: a qualitative study. Sex Relatsh Ther. 2019;34(2):228–41.

Lifestyle Factors Supporting and Maintaining Sexual Activity in Older Adults

11

Sandra Haider, Angela Schwarzinger, and Thomas Ernst Dorner

11.1 Introduction

In older age, sexuality is often a taboo topic or focused on treating sexual dysfunction. Sexuality is seldom seen as something healthy that contributes to one's general well-being. Sex should not only be understood as a pleasurable practice either with a partner or alone, but also within the broader context that includes partnership, trust, physical contact, and intimacy. Scientific evidence clearly shows that sexual activity is closely linked to good health. For example, an Austrian study has shown that dissatisfaction in one's sexual activity and discomfort in one's partnership or in one's family are factors that are most strongly associated with physical symptoms such as joint and muscle pain or subjective decline in strength or endurance [1]. This can be interpreted in two ways: that problems with sexuality or partnership lead to worse health and quality of life, or that physical problems and a lower fitness lead to problems in sexuality and partnership.

Either way, lifestyle factors seem to play an important role and seem to facilitate and modify sexuality. Lifestyle is mostly understood as a behavioural pattern and includes physical activity (PA), diet, smoking habits, and alcohol consumption. In the broader context lifestyle factors are influenced by behavioural factors like personal values, beliefs, personal space, health literacy, sexual orientation, and social factors such as social capital, partnership, or common values and ideologies. In this chapter we focus on classical lifestyle factors and on body weight as direct consequences of PA and nutritional behaviour.

S. Haider (✉) · A. Schwarzinger · T. E. Dorner
Department of Social and Preventive Medicine, Center for Public Health, Medical University of Vienna, Vienna, Austria
e-mail: sandra.a.haider@meduniwien.ac.at; angela@schwarzingers.eu; thomas.dorner@meduniwien.ac.at

11.2 Lifestyle Factors and Sexuality

The association between lifestyle factors and sexuality is depicted in Fig. 11.1. In this figure we hypothesise a causal direction from lifestyle factors that facilitate changes in different levels. The most important classical lifestyle factors are PA, healthy diet, non-smoking or having quit smoking, and adequate alcohol consumption. Those factors are interconnected (e.g. sufficient PA requires non-smoking and a healthy diet) to allow the body to maintain or gain muscle mass.

Optimisation of lifestyle factors leads to positive physiological effects and changes the somatic or mental physiological functions. Lifestyle optimisation can contribute to lower inflammation and better endothelial function and can therefore improve the function of blood vessels and the perfusion of all organs. This is a prerequisite for sexual activity and also improves cardiovascular health. Additionally, lifestyle factors trigger changes in the endocrine and nervous systems. These include

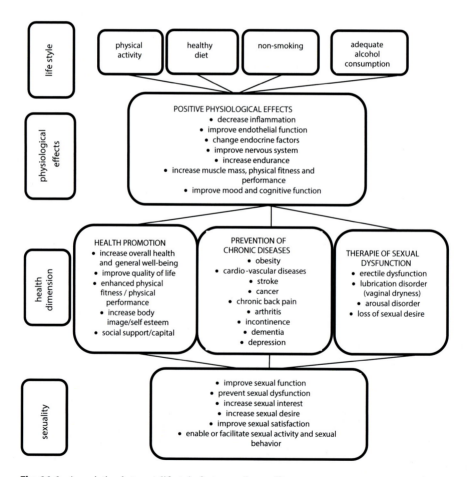

Fig. 11.1 Association between lifestyle factors and sexuality

changes in hormones, neurotransmitters, or immune defence factors like sex hormones, oxytocin, adrenaline, serotonin, or dopamine. The physiological task of these hormones is to prepare for reproduction and to ensure interpersonal bonds. Apart from reproduction, these endocrine factors have positive effects on health such as the anabolic effect on muscles and bones and improved wound healing. They also have a beneficial effect on mental health, including mood and cognitive function. Furthermore, lifestyle factors enhance physical fitness and physical performance, which are beneficial for sexual activity, but also for general health and well-being.

Lifestyle factors influence various health dimensions through which sexuality improves in the following ways:

- Firstly, lifestyle factors increase overall health and well-being on the physical, mental, and social health dimensions. Lifestyle factors increase physical fitness, quality of life, body image, and self-esteem and can increase social capital and social support. All these factors are important for sexuality and show how lifestyle factors improve sexual life.
- Secondly, lifestyle factors contribute towards the prevention of chronic diseases. Some preventable chronic diseases include obesity, cardiovascular diseases, stroke, cancer, chronic back pain, arthritis, incontinence, dementia, or depression. These chronic diseases either physically or mentally lead to sexual dysfunction or decrease sexual interest and sexual desire. Therefore, lifestyle factors that prevent chronic diseases also increase sexual health.
- Thirdly, the ageing process is associated with some changes in men and in women, which influence the sexual function. Some of them are common like erectile dysfunctions (ED) in men or difficulties relating to arousals, orgasm, and lubrication in women [2]. Lifestyle factors can have a direct effect on the function of sexual organs and therefore can contribute to sexual dysfunction therapy.

Summing up, lifestyle optimisation improves sexual function, prevents sexual dysfunction, and increases sexual interest, sexual desire, and sexual satisfaction. Additionally, lifestyle factors enable sexual actions and sexual behaviour. As can be seen, the positive effects of lifestyle factors on sexuality are manifold.

11.2.1 The Lifestyle Factor: Physical Activity

The following pages outline the association of PA with sexuality. Some training methods including practical inputs are subsequently presented.

11.2.1.1 More PA-Better Sexuality/Better Sexuality-More PA

The association between the amount of PA and sexual activities has been shown in some studies. For example, data from the English Longitudinal Study of Ageing, including 3112 people with a mean age of 64.4 (9.8) years, have demonstrated that men doing moderate PA at least once a week have a 1.64 higher chance of having any sexual activity, with a confidence interval (95% CI) of 1.24–2.15 [3]. Also, men doing vigorous PA have an even higher chance of sexual activity, presented by a higher odds ratio (OR) of 2.06 (95% CI: 1.50–2.84). In women performing vigorous PA at least once a week, the chances of being sexually active had an OR of 1.42 (95% CI: 1.09–1.85), which is also higher in comparison to women doing no vigorous PA.

There was also a positive association between fitness levels and frequency of sexual activity, as shown by a cross-sectional study (n = 1039; $\geq$50 years) [4]. In this analysis, 30% of females with the lowest fitness level, 38% with middle fitness, and 66% with the highest fitness level have one or more occasions of sexual intimacy per week. In men, sexual activity was also higher in older adults with better fitness levels, while the corresponding percentages were 46%, 60%, and 63%, respectively. Additionally, a strong positive correlation between fitness levels and degree of sexual satisfaction was seen among men [4].

There are also studies looking at the association between the amount of PA and ED. One of these examinations (n = 3112 men; aged >50 years) has shown that men doing vigorous PA at least once a week had a 0.58 lower chance for ED (95% CI: 0.44–0.77) compared to inactive men [3]. Comparable results have been seen in a cross-sectional analysis including health professionals (n = 31,742 men; age: 53–90) [5].

11.2.1.2 Effects of PA on Sexuality

As stated in the introduction section, it is well proven that regular PA improves overall fitness (aerobic and musculoskeletal capacity), quality of life, mental health, body image, and general well-being [6, 7]. Additionally, regular PA affects the sympathetic nervous system, endocrine factors, and prevents many non-communicable diseases [8]. These positive effects of regular PA can also influence sexuality, as illustrated by the following studies:

- *Quality of life/well-being/enjoyment*: Data have proven that regular PA is related to a better quality of life [7]. This quality of life has also been associated with better sexual function [9]. In a study conducted by Flynn and colleagues on 139 independently living participants with or without a partner (mean age 74 years), a moderately positive correlation was found between quality of life and the frequency and importance of sexual behaviour [9]. Some reasons for the association might be that during sexual activities, endorphins and endogenous opioid peptides are released [10]. Additionally, results of the English Longitudinal Study of Ageing have shown through a four-year follow-up of 2577 men and 3195 women aged $\geq$50 years that men who reported a decline in the frequency of sexual activities had a higher chance for deterioration in self-rated health (OR = 1.47, 95% CI: 1.04–2.08) [11]. In women, a decline in frequency of sexual activities was

also connected with deterioration in self-rated health (OR = 1.64, 95% CI: 1.07–2.51).
- *Longstanding illness*: It is indisputable that PA is a protective factor for chronic illnesses such as type 2 diabetes mellitus, hypertension, obesity, and cardiovascular events [7]. Additionally, PA positively influences low-grade chronic inflammation, whereas the exact mechanism is still unclear [12, 13]. Furthermore, studies have explored an association between longstanding illnesses and sexuality. This association has been shown by the above-mentioned English Longitudinal Study. In this study, men with long-standing illnesses had a higher chance for less sexual activity (OR = 1.69, 95% CI: 1.20–2.37) compared to men with no long-standing illnesses [11]. Another US community-based cross-sectional study including 22,654 people with an age of ≥55 years has found that cancer, bladder/bowel problems, major surgery, poor vision, mental health conditions, cardiovascular diseases, and their risk factors have been related to sexual inactivity [14]. However, poor cardiovascular health has not been shown to be a predictive factor for low sexuality after 5 years (population-based longitudinal investigation n = 1046 men & 1158 women; 57–85 years) [15].
- *Cognitive function*: It has increasingly been shown that regular PA has a positive effect on cognitive function, functional capacity, and dementia [7]. Furthermore, better cognitive function was related to more sexual activities, as shown by Wright and colleagues in a cross-sectional study including 73 participants aged 50–83 years with no history of dementia [16]. A further cross-sectional investigation (n = 6833; 50–89 years) has found significant associations between number sequencing and recall, as well as any form of sexual activity in men, whereas in women only an association between recall and sexual activities was shown [17]. Within the same data set but through a longitudinal design (n = 4476), Smith and colleagues were also able to show that sexually active men at baseline had better immediate and delayed recall over a 4-year follow-up, but no such association was found in women [18].

11.2.1.3 Training Methods
As can be seen from the previous chapter, PA affects many health conditions. Nonetheless, the effects of PA depend on the type of PA (aerobic PA, muscle-strengthening activities, stretching, etc.). For example, aerobic PA has effects on physical endurance whereas muscle-strengthening activities mainly aim at increasing muscle mass. Proven training methods including practical methods that facilitate sexual health are presented below.

Aerobic Physical Activity
Aerobic activities (e.g. Nordic walking, cycling, swimming) make the body's large muscles move in a rhythmic manner for a period of time and cause a person's heart rate to increase [19, 20]. When these activities are performed regularly, aerobic activities have a positive effect on physical endurance measured

by maximum oxygen uptake (VO_{2max}) and make the cardiorespiratory system stronger. Additionally, aerobic activities influence hormones (e.g. testosterone, oestrogen, oxytocin), glucose metabolism, blood pressure, and serum lipid as well as reduce fat mass [20–22]. Older adults doing regular aerobic activities have a reduced risk of age-related loss of physical function [19].

Aerobic training has direct effects on sexual function as well. A systematic review of interventional studies in men with ED (mean age 55 years) revealed that aerobic exercises of 160 min per week over 6 months decreased ED, especially when the ED was caused by physical inactivity, obesity, hypertension, metabolic syndrome, and/or cardiovascular diseases [23]. A reason why PA is especially effective when cardiovascular risk factors are present might be that ED is often a sign of poor vascular function [24]. Another study that included 22 hypertensive men with a mean age of 62.1 years has shown that interval training (60–79% VO_{2max} for 8 weeks duration: 45–60 min/day) reduced ED [25].

In women, literature suggests that aerobic activity at moderate to vigorous intensity has been linked to better sexual arousal, as it increases sympathetic nervous system activity and endocrine factors [8], as well as changes mood through hormone and neurotransmitter levels [26, 27]. Another study ($n = 36$) demonstrated higher vaginal blood circulation and vaginal pulse amplitude after 20 min of ergometer training with 70% of the VO_{2max} when combined with watching an erotic film, compared to just watching an erotic film [27]. However, this study was done in younger women between 18–45 years of age.

Due to these positive effects, it is recommended that older people perform 150 min of moderate or 75 min of vigorous PA or an equivalent combination of both each week. Additional health benefits can be achieved when doing 300 min of moderate intensity activities. If older adults cannot achieve the required amount of activity because of chronic conditions, they should do as much of it as possible [19].

Practical Input

This PA programme follows the actual PA guidelines for older adults [19].

- *Activity*: Aerobic activities can be performed in various ways (e.g. walking, hiking, running, swimming, cycling). Choose the method which seems to be most appropriate for you!
- *Duration*: 150 min of moderate intensity or 75 min of vigorous intensity should be spread through the week.
- *Intensity*: Do moderate or vigorous PA or a combination of both.
    - *Moderate intensity:* Moderate intensity is a level of effort of 5–6 on a scale ranging from 0 to 10, where 0 is the level of sitting, and 10 is maximum effort. A level of 5–6 demands a noticeable increase in breathing and heart rate.
    - *Vigorous intensity:* Vigorous intensity begins at 7 till 8. A level of 7–8 demands a significant increase in breathing and heart rate.

Muscle-Strengthening Exercises and Pelvic Floor Training

Muscle-strengthening exercises (e.g. resistance bands, own body weight, climbing stairs, carrying heavy loads) have substantial effects on various health dimensions and is known to increase skeletal muscle mass, have effects on bone mineral density, glucose metabolism, serum lipids, blood pressure, and basal metabolism [22]. Additionally, muscle-strengthening exercises have effects on sex hormones (testosterone, oestrogens, growth hormone(s), and insulin-like growth factor-1), inducing endogenous hormonal elevations.

As mentioned, muscle-strengthening exercises have a significant effect on muscle mass, which is important when considering that the ageing process is associated with a progressive loss of muscle mass with approximately 30% between 30 and 80 years [28]. This age-related decrease in muscle mass in combination with a loss in muscle strength or function [29], called sarcopenia, is often associated with frailty [30]. Frailty, a geriatric syndrome, is defined as exhaustion, loss of appetite, weakness, functional difficulties, and low PA and is characterised by an increased vulnerability to external stressors [30]. Both sarcopenia and frailty lead to physical disability, dependency, falls, institutionalisation, decreased quality of life, and social isolation [29, 31]. As such, it is obvious that these two phenomena might also influence sexuality in older adults. Consequently, muscle mass and especially muscle strength is a key factor in maintaining functional independence in older adults.

When thinking of sexual function, strengthening the pelvic floor muscle (PFM) seems of special importance as its strength, power, and endurance are important for maintaining urinary continence and may have benefits for sexual satisfaction [32]. For example, in a multicentre study of middle-aged women (n = 585 women, 54.9 years) a strong pelvic floor was a predictor for sexual activities, and women with a strong pelvic floor had a 1.89 higher chance of engaging in sexual activities (OR = 1.89, 95 CI: 1.18–3.03). It has also been shown that pelvic floor training resulted in a reduction in problems with their sex lives [33]. In this context it must be mentioned that urinary incontinence is a factor affecting sexual desire and satisfaction [34]. Dissatisfaction with sexual life was strongly correlated to worries about urinary leakage during intercourse (n = 147; 18–74 years) [35]. Based on data from a Cochrane systematic review including 31 trials (n = 1817 women), PFM training can cure or improve symptoms of all types of urinary incontinence. It may reduce the number of leakage episodes and the quantity of leakage, consequently improving the quality of life [36]. In men, evidence suggests that the pelvic floor muscles play a crucial role in penile rigidity [37]. A systematic review (7 studies, 478 participants; 43–69 years) has revealed that PFM training in combination with aerobic activities improves patient-reported erectile function [26]. The findings of PFM training and its association with sexuality were mainly from younger populations. Nonetheless, the PFM training method could also be applied for older people.

Addressing frailty and sarcopenia, it is recommended to do muscle-strengthening activities of moderate or higher intensity for the major muscle groups, two or more days a week [19]. Additionally, strengthening the pelvic floor muscles might improve sexual activity in older adults.

Practical Input for Muscle-Strengthening in General
This PA programme followed the actual PA guidelines for older adults [19].

- *Activities*: Muscle-strengthening exercises can be performed in various ways (e.g. weight-lifting; elastic bands, own body weight). Choose the method which seems to be most appropriate for you!
- *Frequency*: The major muscle groups (legs, hips, back, abdomen, chest, shoulders, and arms) should be trained at least 2 days a week.
- *Sets and repetitions*: Do 1–3 sets of 8–12 repetitions for each exercise.
- *Intensity*: Exercises should be performed to a point at which it is difficult to do another repetition.

Practical Input for Pelvic Floor Training Based on Olliver [38]
- *Activity*
  - Lying down, stomach and thigh muscles are relaxed. Focus on PFM. (Squeeze the PFM and lift them inside up. Imagine an open flower, which closes.)
  - Contract PFM for 5 s and relax.
  - Repeat it 10 times.
- *Frequency*
  - Week 1: 10 cycles, 3 times.
  - Week 2–5: increase up to 50 cycles, 3 times.
  - Maintain 30 consecutive cycles daily.

Stretching

Stretching exercises lengthen shortened tissue and enhance the ability of joints to move through their full range of motion. They also relax hypertonic muscles and thus allow older adults to perform daily activities more easily. Since improved flexibility reduces the risk of injury, older adults should maintain their flexibility, making stretching exercises part of their PA programme [19].

When thinking about sexuality, flexibility might also play a relevant role, especially in older age. However, to the authors' knowledge there has been no study investigating the effect of stretching exercises alone. However, research has investigated the effectiveness of combined psycho-physiological therapy, including stretching and breathing exercises, as a new alternative therapy for sexual satisfaction. In this context one study was found in middle-aged heterosexual men, married for a minimum of 6 months, and recruited in a hospital ($n = 80$ men; 20–55 years). The study showed that men who practiced combined psycho-physiological therapy including stretching and breathing for 20 sessions with a duration of 90–120 min had improved sexual satisfaction, whereas the intervention group did not have significantly better scores than the control group continuing their daily routine [36]. Looking at the intervention in detail, each session started with a 10-min warm-up, followed by rhythmic breathing and a stretching therapy while each muscle was stretched separately. Each lesson was finished by rhythmic breathing.

Summing up, there are only single studies with small sample sizes of younger people looking at the effect of stretching on sexuality. Hence, no clear recommendation can be given at this point. However, when bearing the above-mentioned general benefits in mind, it might be hypothesised that stretching can positively affect sexuality in older adults. Therefore, some practical input is given below.

Practical Input
- *Stretching and breathing* based on Bay et al. [36].
  - Start rhythmic breathing as a warm-up to harmonise the body and mind. You can use the following breathing technique: Breath slowly and deep four times per minute.
  - Then stretch muscle slowly and passively for the full range of motion. The major muscle groups should be stretched.
  - For maximum gain, remain in stretching position for about 20–30 s or until the muscle relaxes.
  - Exhale when a muscle is stretched; inhale when a muscle is relaxed.
  - Finish session with rhythmic breathing.
  - Note: It is important to take time, breath, and relax; therefore a session of 60–90 min is advised.

Yoga

Yoga—literally meaning "union"—might be another facilitator to healthy sexuality, also in older adults. Yoga comprises aerobic training, muscle strengthening, mindfulness exercises, and stretching, depending on the type of yoga and the practiced postures. Additionally, yoga includes breathing exercises [32, 36].

Generally the health effects of yoga have been proven on multiple physical function outcomes in older adults such as strength, balance, flexibility, and mental well-being [33]. Consequently, authors demanded the addition of yoga to the PA guidelines for older adults.

Concerning the impact of yoga on sexual health, research is limited. One pilot study was found where sexually active young men with no clinical diagnosis participated in a 12-week yoga camp doing Yoga Asanas ($n = 65$; 40 (8.3) years) [34]. Results showed a significant improvement in sexual function measured by the Male Sexual Quotient (before: 66.4 (10.9); after: 78.2 (6.1)). The same authors performed the same intervention in healthy women ($n = 40$; 34.7 (8.5) years). The participants were also able to improve sexual function, measured by the Female Sexual Function Index (before: 23.7 (8.5); after: 30.4 (3.1).

To sum up, the effects of yoga on the general health of the elderly population have been proven. However, studies looking at the effect of yoga on sexual health are missing to a great extent. When bearing the above-mentioned general health benefits in mind, it might be hypothesised that yoga can positively affect sexuality in older adults.

> **Take-Home Message**
> To sum up the literature concerning PA, studies suggest to perform…
>
> - … *aerobic exercises* for 150 min of moderate intensity or 75 min of vigorous intensity or an equivalent combination of both every week.
> - … *muscle-strengthening* exercises with moderate or greater intensity involving the major muscle groups for two or more days a week. When thinking of sexual health, strengthening the pelvic floor muscle seems of special importance.
> - … *stretching exercises* of the major muscle groups.
> - As *yoga* has been shown to improve physical functioning in older adults, it might be hypothesised that yoga can improve their sexual health as well. However, studies are broadly missing.

11.2.2 Lifestyle Factor: Healthy Diet

A healthy diet is another lifestyle factor which influences the sexual behaviour of older adults. As mentioned before the prevention of sarcopenia and frailty in the older population plays a role, as these factors are relevant to maintain mobility and avoid independency. There is also a body of studies looking at various diets and nutritional supplements which might influence overall health and sexual activity as well. An overview of the potential effect of nutritional habits is given above.

11.2.2.1 Sarcopenia and Protein Intake

Sarcopenia is a major problem associated with the ageing process. Based on the definition of the "European Working Group on Sarcopenia in Older People" sarcopenia is the age-related decrease in muscle mass in combination with a loss in muscle strength or function [29]. This decline in muscle mass comes up to approximately 30% between the age of 30 and 80 years [28]. Additionally, muscle strength decreases significantly, making up a decrease of 20–40% in men and 50% in women older than 80 years [35]. Sarcopenia and geriatric syndrome frailty [30] are associated with an increased risk of falls, fractures, cardiovascular disease, dependence, hospitalisation, and all-cause mortality [29, 39]. Due to these serious health outcomes, sarcopenia and frailty should be avoided [37], a consequence of which sexual ability can be maintained.

Modifiable factors that can prevent sarcopenia and frailty are enough PA and a healthy diet, whereas special attention should be paid to protein intake [29, 40]. As such, a protein intake for at least 1.0–1.2 g/kg body weight/day is suggested for healthy older adults [41–43]. For older adults with acute or chronic illnesses, 1.2–1.5 g/kg body weight/day may be indicated. In some publications up to 2.0 g/kg body weight/day are recommended and should be individually adjusted depending on the nutritional status, PA level, disease status, and tolerance [43, 44].

Summing up, the nutritional recommendations for older adults should be achieved to avoid an excessive loss of muscle mass, which can lead to restrictions in daily life and reduced sexual ability.

11.2.2.2 Fruits and Vegetables/Mediterranean Diet

According to the above-mentioned nutritional recommendations, the diet should also be rich in fruits and vegetables, where variety is as important as quantity [45]. This diet was shown to reduce blood pressure and the risk of cardiovascular disease, as well as prevent some types of cancer and premature mortality [46, 47].

There are also studies looking at the direct effect of fruits and vegetable intake on sexual function. In a longitudinal study of 1564 men older than ≥65 years, recruited in housing estates and community centres, it has been shown that high levels of fruits and vegetable consumption (>350 g/1000 kcal/day) were associated with a reduced International Prostate Symptoms Scale, but not with less ED or sexual activities after 4 years [48].

Concerning various diet styles the Mediterranean diet, which is rich in fruits, vegetables, whole grain, legumes, walnut, and olive oil, was shown to improve physical performance and to protect against muscle wasting [49]. As it also reduces cardiovascular risk factors, cognitive decline, the risk for breast cancer, and all-cause mortality, it was recommended for menopausal women [50].

Additionally, a systematic review including observational and interventional studies has shown that ED was less prevalent in men sticking to the Mediterranean-style diet compared to men with the Western diet [51]. The fact that the Mediterranean diet is a protective factor for ED was also confirmed by a recent review [52]. Additionally, a Mediterranean diet in combination with regular exercise can even help to regain sexual activity [53]. In women with obesity, diabetes, or metabolic syndrome, the same diet was also shown to increase sexual function, alleviate sexual dysfunction, change metabolic markers, and reduce inflammatory cytokines [54].

To sum up, while one's fruit and vegetable intake is relevant to absorbing sufficient micronutrients, the literature suggests adhering to a Mediterranean diet style.

11.2.2.3 Supplements

In addition to a balanced diet, there are also supplements which might facilitate sexual activity in two ways. While supplements are relevant to avoid malnutrition and sarcopenia and to enhance one's health status, they directly influence sexual function.

In general, current evidence does not support routine supplementation for well-nourished older people [55]. Older adults should eat food with high energy density and achieve the nutritional recommendations whenever possible. However, when wanting to prevent malnutrition and sarcopenia, supplements might be used to avoid or minimise functional limitations and to maintain physical function [43, 55], as a consequence of which sexual activity can be improved or maintained. As mentioned before the uptake of proteins is especially relevant in this age group.

There are also studies looking at the effect of supplements on sexual function per se. In the majority of these studies supplements are used as a therapy to treat ED. Micronutrients are potentially important for sex hormone synthesis, particularly during the age-related decline in the endocrine system [37]. A systematic review has looked at the effect of these micronutrients on the hormone system. Authors have found no significant effects of micronutrients (vitamins A, C, D, or E; carotenoids; iron; copper; zinc; magnesium; selenium; and potassium) on sex hormones. However, authors have stated that the data are limited and that the included trials have significant methodological limitations [37].

It has also been discussed that amino acids can positively influence sexuality. Theoretically, L-arginine helps the blood vessels to relax and to promote good blood flow by using nitrous oxide. L-citrulline is another amino acid, which is converted to L-arginine. As studies have shown that patients with ED have low L-arginine and L-citrulline level, increased levels might reduce problems [56]. The recent systematic review and meta-analysis of Rhim et al. [57] has concluded that L-arginine supplements should be recommended to patients with mild to moderate ED. However, they have stated that the dosage and the duration vary among studies, making the conclusion limited. This was confirmed by Koolwal and colleagues [58]. There are also studies stating that there is no scientific evidence for L-arginine [59]. Compared to L-arginine there are only some small studies of L-citrulline making a recommendation of its effects even more difficult [60].

Panax ginseng is another frequently used product for ED [61]. The physiological effect is that Panax ginseng may increase NO and reduce homocysteine at the same time [62]. Although a systematic review and meta-analysis has showed a possible effect on ED, a definite answer to this is needed through further studies with larger sample sizes [63].

Summing up, there is no scientific evidence that directly supports the effects of supplements (micronutrient, amino acid, panax ginseng) on sexual function. However, supplements can operate indirectly, when they are used to avoid sarcopenia, malnutrition, or frailty.

Take-Home Message
Studies suggest…

- … to meet the nutritional recommendations for the healthy elderly.
- … to have a protein intake of at least 1.0–2.0 g/kg body weight/day.
- … to have an adequate energy intake rich in nutrients.
- … no clear recommendations can be given for supplements.

11.2.3 Lifestyle Factor: Alcohol

Alcohol consumption is associated with various short- and long-term health risks including high blood pressure, liver disease, and various cancers (e.g. breast cancer) among others, whereas the risk of these harms increases with intake [64]. In this context it has to be considered that recent studies question the protective health benefits (e.g. reducing risk of heart disease) of even moderate alcohol consumption [65]. Additionally, it has to be taken into account that alcohol contains a lot of calories, which can increase body weight.

When looking at the direct effect of alcohol on women's sexual functions, literature indicates opposing views [66]. On the one hand there are studies that show no effect of alcohol on sexual arousal, pleasure, or orgasm, while on the other, investigations show positive effects. Additionally, it was shown that older women who frequently drink alcohol perceived sex as more important, and have sex-related discussions with a physician more often. To this, higher risky sexual behaviours and a higher prevalence of depression are mentioned as possible reasons [66].

In men, studies suggest that alcohol consumption and sexual function are associated in a J-shaped manner, where moderate alcohol consumption has a protective effect on ED [67]. This is confirmed by a further prospective cohort study in the general population ($n = 31{,}742$ men; age: 53–90) [5]. Moderate alcohol consumption was also a protective factor for ED in diabetic men, treated in 26 diabetes clinics in Israel ($n = 1040$; mean age 57 years; OR: 0.7; 95%CI: 0.51–0.97) [68]. Additionally, a cross-sectional study ($n = 1.580$ men, >20 years) has shown that current drinkers have a 25–30% reduced probability for ED [69]. Authors assume that these beneficial effects may be due to the long-term effects of high-density lipoprotein cholesterol and other variables, leading to a higher bioavailability of NO [70]. Of note, literature generally agrees that out of control drinking has negative effects, as behaviour and relationships with other people are affected. Consequently, it is recommended to avoid excessive alcohol consumption for good erectile function, where one to two drinks have been mentioned as the maximum amount to be consumed per day (level B evidence) [70].

> **Take-Home Message**
> Studies suggest…
>
> - … none to moderate alcohol consumption facilitates good sexual function and sexual satisfaction.

11.2.4 Lifestyle Factor: Non-smoking

It is well known that smoking is one of the leading preventable causes of death, as it represents a great risk for cardiovascular diseases, stroke, and lung diseases (e.g. COPD, asthma, cancer), affecting a person's overall health [71, 72]. As such and when bearing in mind that longstanding illnesses are associated with worse sexual function, non-smoking has positive effects on sexuality.

Additionally, there is a positive effect of non-smoking and ED, when compared to direct and second-hand smoking exposure [73, 74]. For example, a meta-analysis of four prospective cohort studies has shown that the risk for ED was 51% higher in current smokers, and 20% higher in ex-smokers compared with people who never smoked [75]. There are also examinations assessing the effects of smoking cessation, showing that cessation significantly enhanced both physiological and self-reported indices of sexual health, irrespective of baseline ED [76]. The positive effect of smoking cessation was also confirmed by Pourmand and colleagues, who recruited smokers ($n = 281$; aged 30–60 years) requesting nicotine replacement therapy and who complained about ED [77]. In this study ED status improved in 25% of ex-smokers but in none of the current smokers after 1 year of follow-up.

As smoking is one of the leading preventable causes of death and literature also revealed a direct effect on ED, smoking cessation is suggested to maintain sexual satisfaction [70].

> **Take-Home Message**
> Studies suggest…
>
> - … to remain a non-smoker or to quit smoking.

11.2.5 Lifestyle Factor: Body Weight

As mentioned in the introduction, PA and healthy diet influence body weight, having effects on various health dimensions and as a consequence influencing sexuality. In older adults in general, a body weight of 23.0–29.9 kg/m^2 is recommended, as it is associated with the lowest all-cause mortality [78]. As such, in older adults a BMI typically categorised as "overweight" is not related to adverse mortality outcomes [79]. However, obesity is associated with an increased risk for non-communicable diseases and should therefore be avoided [80].

Exploring the association between body weight and sexual activity, results of the population-representative English Longitudinal Study of Ageing ($n = 2220$ men & 2737 women; mean age 68.2 years) have showed that men with overweight had a 1.45 higher probability of engaging in sexual activities, with a confidence interval of 1.15–1.81 compared to men with normal weight. Also, men with obesity had a higher chance of engaging in sexual activities (OR = 1.38, 95% CI: 1.07–1.77) than those with normal weight [81]. In women, the results were comparable in that women with overweight had a higher chance of engaging in sexual intercourse (OR = 1.34, 95% CI: 1.05–1.71) compared to women with normal weight.

However, there are studies on the association between body weight and sexual dysfunction revealing that obesity is associated with ED. For example results of a review reported a 30–90% higher risk in overweight or men with overweight or obesity [82]. This might be due to the fact that obesity and ED share similar pathological pathways [83]. The same above-mentioned review has summarised that women with metabolic syndrome have an increased prevalence for sexual dysfunction as compared with women with normal weight [82]. However, these results do not especially apply to older adults.

From the results of longitudinal studies, the Health Professionals Follow-up Study including 31,724 men free of ED at baseline (age 53–90 years) deserves mention. This investigation has revealed that men with a BMI >28.7 kg/m^2 had a 1.3 higher relative risk (95% Cl: 1.2–1.4) for developing ED than men with a BMI <23.2 kg/m^2 after 2 years [5]. In a further study, authors reported a 70–96% higher probability for developing ED in men with obesity compared to men with normal weight with follow-up between 5 and 25 years [70]. As such, in older men with obesity a negative energy balance through increasing PA and reducing energy intake might be an effective intervention for ED, as it reduces body weight, which also reduces pro-inflammatory state and the available NO [84, 85].

Summing up, despite having a higher chance of engaging in sexual activity, obesity in older adults should be avoided to prevent chronic disease and sexual dysfunction through following a healthy diet and enough PA.

11.3 Summary

As can be seen from the cited studies, a healthy lifestyle consisting of an adequate amount of PA, a healthy diet, the absence of smoking, and none to moderate alcohol consumption can be seen to facilitate better sexuality in older adults. This lifestyle has positive physiological effects and influences health in various dimensions, improving general health, preventing chronic diseases, as well as preventing sexual dysfunctions.

References

1. Dorner TE, Stronegger WJ, Rebhandl E, Rieder A, Freidl W. The relationship between various psychosocial factors and physical symptoms reported during primary-care health examinations. Wien Klin Wochenschr. 2010;122(3–4):103–9. https://doi.org/10.1007/s00508-010-1312-6.
2. Lee DM, Nazroo J, O'Connor DB, Blake M, Pendleton N. Sexual health and well-being among older men and women in England: findings from the English longitudinal study of ageing. Arch Sex Behav. 2016;45(1):133–44. https://doi.org/10.1007/s10508-014-0465-1.
3. Smith L, Grabovac I, Yang L, Veronese N, Koyanagi A, Jackson SE. Participation in physical activity is associated with sexual activity in older English adults. Int J Environ Res Public Health. 2019;16(3):489. https://doi.org/10.3390/ijerph16030489.
4. Bortz WM 2nd, Wallace DH. Physical fitness, aging, and sexuality. West J Med. 1999;170(3):167–9.
5. Bacon CG, Mittleman MA, Kawachi I, Giovannucci E, Glasser DB, Rimm EB. Sexual function in men older than 50 years of age: results from the health professionals follow-up study. Ann Intern Med. 2003;139(3):161–8. https://doi.org/10.7326/0003-4819-139-3-200308050-00005.

6. Langhammer B, Bergland A, Rydwik E. The importance of physical activity exercise among older people. Biomed Res Int. 2018;2018:7856823. https://doi.org/10.1155/2018/7856823.
7. Bauman A, Merom D, Bull FC, Buchner DM, Fiatarone Singh MA. Updating the evidence for physical activity: summative reviews of the epidemiological evidence, prevalence, and interventions to promote "active aging". Gerontologist. 2016;56(Suppl 2):268–80. https://doi.org/10.1093/geront/gnw031.
8. Stanton AM, Handy AB, Meston CM. The effects of exercise on sexual function in women. Sex Med Rev. 2018;6(4):548–57. https://doi.org/10.1016/j.sxmr.2018.02.004.
9. Flynn TJ, Gow AJ. Examining associations between sexual behaviours and quality of life in older adults. Age Ageing. 2015;44(5):823–8. https://doi.org/10.1093/ageing/afv083.
10. Darko DF, Irwin MR, Risch SC, Gillin JC. Plasma beta-endorphin and natural killer cell activity in major depression: a preliminary study. Psychiatry Res. 1992;43(2):111–9. https://doi.org/10.1016/0165-1781(92)90125-m.
11. Jackson SE, Yang L, Koyanagi A, Stubbs B, Veronese N, Smith L. Declines in sexual activity and function predict incident health problems in older adults: prospective findings from the English longitudinal study of ageing. Arch Sex Behav. 2020;49(3):929–40. https://doi.org/10.1007/s10508-019-1443-4.
12. Haider SL, Grabovac I, Winzer E, Kapan A, Schindler KE, Lackinger C, Titze S, Dorner TE. Change in inflammatory parameters in prefrail and frail persons obtaining physical training and nutritional support international conference of frailty and sarcopenia. Barcelona 2017.
13. Franceschi C, Garagnani P, Parini P, Giuliani C, Santoro A. Inflammaging: a new immune-metabolic viewpoint for age-related diseases. Nat Rev Endocrinol. 2018;14(10):576–90. https://doi.org/10.1038/s41574-018-0059-4.
14. Bach LE, Mortimer JA, VandeWeerd C, Corvin J. The association of physical and mental health with sexual activity in older adults in a retirement community. J Sex Med. 2013;10(11):2671–8. https://doi.org/10.1111/jsm.12308.
15. Liu H, Waite LJ, Shen S, Wang DH. Is sex good for your health? A national study on partnered sexuality and cardiovascular risk among older men and women. J Health Soc Behav. 2016;57(3):276–96. https://doi.org/10.1177/0022146516661597.
16. Wright H, Jenks RA, Demeyere N. Frequent sexual activity predicts specific cognitive abilities in older adults. J Gerontol B Psychol Sci Soc Sci. 2019;74(1):47–51. https://doi.org/10.1093/geronb/gbx065.
17. Wright H, Jenks RA. Sex on the brain! Associations between sexual activity and cognitive function in older age. Age Ageing. 2016;45(2):313–7. https://doi.org/10.1093/ageing/afv197.
18. Smith L, Grabovac I, Yang L, Lopez-Sanchez GF, Firth J, Pizzol D, et al. Sexual activity and cognitive decline in older age: a prospective cohort study. Aging Clin Exp Res. 2020;32(1):85–91. https://doi.org/10.1007/s40520-019-01334-z.
19. US Department of Health and Human Services. Physical activity guidelines for Americans. 2nd ed. Washington, DC: U.S. Department of Health and Human Services; 2018.
20. Moghetti P, Bacchi E, Brangani C, Donà S, Negri C. Metabolic effects of exercise. Front Horm Res. 2016;47:44–57. https://doi.org/10.1159/000445156.
21. Braith RW, Stewart KJ. Resistance exercise training: its role in the prevention of cardiovascular disease. Circulation. 2006;113(22):2642–50.
22. Pollock ML, Franklin BA, Balady GJ, Chaitman BL, Fleg JL, Fletcher B, et al. AHA Science Advisory. Resistance exercise in individuals with and without cardiovascular disease: benefits, rationale, safety, and prescription: an advisory from the Committee on Exercise, Rehabilitation, and Prevention, Council on Clinical Cardiology, American Heart Association; Position paper endorsed by the American College of Sports Medicine. Circulation. 2000;101(7):828–33. https://doi.org/10.1161/01.cir.101.7.828.
23. Gerbild H, Larsen CM, Graugaard C, Areskoug JK. Physical activity to improve erectile function: a systematic review of intervention studies. Sex Med. 2018;6(2):75–89. https://doi.org/10.1016/j.esxm.2018.02.001.

24. Silva AB, Sousa N, Azevedo LF, Martins C. Physical activity and exercise for erectile dysfunction: systematic review and meta-analysis. Br J Sports Med. 2017;51(19):1419–24. https://doi.org/10.1136/bjsports-2016-096418.
25. Lamina S, Okoye CG, Dagogo TT. Therapeutic effect of an interval exercise training program in the management of erectile dysfunction in hypertensive patients. J Clin Hypertens. 2009;11(3):125–9. https://doi.org/10.1111/j.1751-7176.2009.00086.x.
26. Meston CM, Gorzalka BB. The effects of sympathetic activation on physiological and subjective sexual arousal in women. Behav Res Ther. 1995;33(6):651–64. https://doi.org/10.1016/0005-7967(95)00006-j.
27. Meston CM, Gorzalka BB. Differential effects of sympathetic activation on sexual arousal in sexually dysfunctional and functional women. J Abnorm Psychol. 1996;105(4):582–91. https://doi.org/10.1037//0021-843x.105.4.582.
28. Frontera WR, Hughes VA, Fielding RA, Fiatarone MA, Evans WJ, Roubenoff R. Aging of skeletal muscle: a 12-yr longitudinal study. J Appl Physiol (1985). 2000;88(4):1321–6. https://doi.org/10.1152/jappl.2000.88.4.1321.
29. Cruz-Jentoft AJ, Baeyens JP, Bauer JM, Boirie Y, Cederholm T, Landi F, et al. Sarcopenia: European consensus on definition and diagnosis: report of the European working group on sarcopenia in older people. Age Ageing. 2010;39(4):412–23. https://doi.org/10.1093/ageing/afq034.
30. Fried LP, Tangen CM, Walston J, Newman AB, Hirsch C, Gottdiener J, et al. Frailty in older adults: evidence for a phenotype. J Gerontol A Biol Sci Med Sci. 2001;56(3):M146–56.
31. Clegg A, Young J, Iliffe S, Rikkert MO, Rockwood K. Frailty in elderly people. Lancet. 2013;381(9868):752–62. https://doi.org/10.1016/s0140-6736(12)62167-9.
32. Brotto LA, Krychman M, Jacobson P. Eastern approaches for enhancing women's sexuality: mindfulness, acupuncture, and yoga (CME). J Sex Med. 2008;5(12):2741–8; quiz 9. https://doi.org/10.1111/j.1743-6109.2008.01071.x.
33. Sivaramakrishnan D, Fitzsimons C, Kelly P, Ludwig K, Mutrie N, Saunders DH, et al. The effects of yoga compared to active and inactive controls on physical function and health related quality of life in older adults- systematic review and meta-analysis of randomised controlled trials. Int J Behav Nutr Phys Act. 2019;16(1):33. https://doi.org/10.1186/s12966-019-0789-2.
34. Dhikav V, Karmarkar G, Verma M, Gupta R, Gupta S, Mittal D, et al. Yoga in male sexual functioning: a noncompararive pilot study. J Sex Med. 2010;7(10):3460–6. https://doi.org/10.1111/j.1743-6109.2010.01930.x.
35. Doherty TJ. Invited review: aging and sarcopenia. J Appl Physiol. 2003;95(4):1717–27. https://doi.org/10.1152/japplphysiol.00347.2003.
36. Bay R, Ismail SB, Zahiruddin WM, Arifin WN. Effect of combined psycho-physiological stretching and breathing therapy on sexual satisfaction. BMC Urol. 2013;13:16. https://doi.org/10.1186/1471-2490-13-16.
37. Janjuha R, Bunn D, Hayhoe R, Hooper L, Abdelhamid A, Mahmood S, et al. Effects of dietary or supplementary micronutrients on sex hormones and IGF-1 in middle and older age: a systematic review and meta-analysis. Nutrients. 2020;12(5):1457. https://doi.org/10.3390/nu12051457.
38. Olliver J. The best exercises for Sex [19.10.2020]. https://www.academia.edu/35686093/Specific_Exercise_for_the_Treatment_of_Erectile_Dysfunction_and_Premature_Ejaculation.
39. Fried LP, Ferrucci L, Darer J, Williamson JD, Anderson G. Untangling the concepts of disability, frailty, and comorbidity: implications for improved targeting and care. J Gerontol A Biol Sci Med Sci. 2004;59(3):255–63.
40. Lang PO, Michel JP, Zekry D. Frailty syndrome: a transitional state in a dynamic process. Gerontology. 2009;55(5):539–49. https://doi.org/10.1159/000211949.
41. Tessier AJ, Chevalier S. An update on protein, leucine, omega-3 fatty acids, and vitamin D in the prevention and treatment of sarcopenia and functional decline. Nutrients. 2018;10(8):1099. https://doi.org/10.3390/nu10081099.

42. Deutz NE, Bauer JM, Barazzoni R, Biolo G, Boirie Y, Bosy-Westphal A, et al. Protein intake and exercise for optimal muscle function with aging: recommendations from the ESPEN Expert Group. Clin Nutr. 2014;33(6):929–36. https://doi.org/10.1016/j.clnu.2014.04.007.
43. Volkert D, Beck AM, Cederholm T, Cruz-Jentoft A, Goisser S, Hooper L, et al. ESPEN guideline on clinical nutrition and hydration in geriatrics. Clin Nutr. 2019;38(1):10–47. https://doi.org/10.1016/j.clnu.2018.05.024.
44. Paddon-Jones D, Short KR, Campbell WW, Volpi E, Wolfe RR. Role of dietary protein in the sarcopenia of aging. Am J Clin Nutr. 2008;87(5):1562S–6S. https://doi.org/10.1093/ajcn/87.5.1562S.
45. University of Harvard. Healthy eating plate. [19 July 2013]. www.hsph.harvard.edu/nutritionsource/healthy-eating-plate/.
46. Wang X, Ouyang Y, Liu J, Zhu M, Zhao G, Bao W, et al. Fruit and vegetable consumption and mortality from all causes, cardiovascular disease, and cancer: systematic review and dose-response meta-analysis of prospective cohort studies. BMJ. 2014;349:g4490. https://doi.org/10.1136/bmj.g4490.
47. Aune D, Keum N, Giovannucci E, Fadnes LT, Boffetta P, Greenwood DC, et al. Dietary intake and blood concentrations of antioxidants and the risk of cardiovascular disease, total cancer, and all-cause mortality: a systematic review and dose-response meta-analysis of prospective studies. Am J Clin Nutr. 2018;108(5):1069–91. https://doi.org/10.1093/ajcn/nqy097.
48. Liu ZM, Wong CK, Chan D, Tse LA, Yip B, Wong SY. Fruit and vegetable intake in relation to lower urinary tract symptoms and erectile dysfunction among southern Chinese elderly men: a 4-year prospective study of Mr OS Hong Kong. Medicine. 2016;95(4):e2557. https://doi.org/10.1097/MD.0000000000002557.
49. Ganapathy A, Nieves JW. Nutrition and Sarcopenia-what do we know? Nutrients. 2020;12(6):1755. https://doi.org/10.3390/nu12061755.
50. Cano A, Marshall S, Zolfaroli I, Bitzer J, Ceausu I, Chedraui P, et al. The Mediterranean diet and menopausal health: an EMAS position statement. Maturitas. 2020;139:90–7. https://doi.org/10.1016/j.maturitas.2020.07.001.
51. Esposito K, Giugliano F, Maiorino MI, Giugliano D. Dietary factors, Mediterranean diet and erectile dysfunction. J Sex Med. 2010;7(7):2338–45. https://doi.org/10.1111/j.1743-6109.2010.01842.x.
52. La J, Roberts NH, Yafi FA. Diet and Men's sexual health. Sex Med Rev. 2018;6(1):54–68. https://doi.org/10.1016/j.sxmr.2017.07.004.
53. Giugliano D, Giugliano F, Esposito K. Sexual dysfunction and the Mediterranean diet. Public Health Nutr. 2006;9(8A):1118–20. https://doi.org/10.1017/S1368980007668542.
54. Towe M, La J, El-Khatib F, Roberts N, Yafi FA, Rubin R. Diet and female sexual health. Sex Med Rev. 2020;8(2):256–64. https://doi.org/10.1016/j.sxmr.2019.08.004.
55. Milne AC, Avenell A, Potter J. Meta-analysis: protein and energy supplementation in older people. Ann Intern Med. 2006;144(1):37–48. https://doi.org/10.7326/0003-4819-144-1-200601030-00008.
56. Barassi A, Corsi Romanelli MM, Pezzilli R, Damele CA, Vaccalluzzo L, Goi G, et al. Levels of l-arginine and l-citrulline in patients with erectile dysfunction of different etiology. Andrology. 2017;5(2):256–61. https://doi.org/10.1111/andr.12293.
57. Rhim HC, Kim MS, Park YJ, Choi WS, Park HK, Kim HG, et al. The potential role of arginine supplements on erectile dysfunction: a systemic review and meta-analysis. J Sex Med. 2019;16(2):223–34. https://doi.org/10.1016/j.jsxm.2018.12.002.
58. Koolwal A, Manohar JS, Rao TSS, Koolwal GD. L-arginine and erectile dysfunction. J Psychosex Health. 2019;1(1):37–43. https://doi.org/10.1177/2631831818822018.
59. Haensch CA DGfN. Diagnostik und Therapie der erektilen Dysfunktion, S1-Leitlinie. 2018.
60. Cormio L, De Siati M, Lorusso F, Selvaggio O, Mirabella L, Sanguedolce F, et al. Oral L-citrulline supplementation improves erection hardness in men with mild erectile dysfunction. Urology. 2011;77(1):119–22. https://doi.org/10.1016/j.urology.2010.08.028.
61. Balasubramanian A, Thirumavalavan N, Srivatsav A, Yu J, Hotaling JM, Lipshultz LI, et al. An analysis of popular online erectile dysfunction supplements. J Sex Med. 2019;16(6):843–52. https://doi.org/10.1016/j.jsxm.2019.03.269.

62. Pyke RE. Toward a scientific nutritional supplement combination for Prostatism and erectile dysfunction I: from known pharmacology to clinical testing. J Med Food. 2019;22(5):529–37. https://doi.org/10.1089/jmf.2018.0148.
63. Borrelli F, Colalto C, Delfino DV, Iriti M, Izzo AA. Herbal dietary supplements for erectile dysfunction: a systematic review and meta-analysis. Drugs. 2018;78(6):643–73. https://doi.org/10.1007/s40265-018-0897-3.
64. Prevention; CfDCa. Alcohol use and your health.
65. Prevention; CfDCa. Alcohol and public health.
66. Bergeron CD, Goltz HH, Szucs LE, Reyes JV, Wilson KL, Ory MG, et al. Exploring sexual behaviors and health communication among older women. Health Care Women Int. 2017;38(12):1356–72. https://doi.org/10.1080/07399332.2017.1329308.
67. Cheng JY, Ng EM, Chen RY, Ko JS. Alcohol consumption and erectile dysfunction: meta-analysis of population-based studies. Int J Impot Res. 2007;19(4):343–52. https://doi.org/10.1038/sj.ijir.3901556.
68. Kalter-Leibovici O, Wainstein J, Ziv A, Harman-Bohem I, Murad H, Raz I. Clinical, socioeconomic, and lifestyle parameters associated with erectile dysfunction among diabetic men. Diabetes Care. 2005;28(7):1739–44. https://doi.org/10.2337/diacare.28.7.1739.
69. Chew KK. Alcohol consumption and male erectile dysfunction: an unfounded reputation for risk? J Sex Med. 2009;6(8):2340. https://doi.org/10.1111/j.1743-6109.2009.01333.x.
70. Maiorino MI, Bellastella G, Esposito K. Lifestyle modifications and erectile dysfunction: what can be expected? Asian J Androl. 2015;17(1):5–10. https://doi.org/10.4103/1008-682X.137687.
71. Services UDoHaH. The health consequences of smoking—50 years of progress: a report of the surgeon general - a report of the surgeon general. Atlanta, GA: Centers for Disease Control and Prevention (US); 2014.
72. Services UDoHaH. How tobacco smoke causes disease: what it means to you. Atlanta: U.S. Department of Health and Human Services, Centers for Disease Control and Prevention, National Center for Chronic Disease Prevention and Health Promotion, Office on Smoking and Health; 2010.
73. Kupelian V, Link CL, McKinlay JB. Association between smoking, passive smoking, and erectile dysfunction: results from the Boston Area Community Health (BACH) Survey. Eur Urol. 2007;52(2):416–22. https://doi.org/10.1016/j.eururo.2007.03.015.
74. Polsky JY, Aronson KJ, Heaton JP, Adams MA. Smoking and other lifestyle factors in relation to erectile dysfunction. BJU Int. 2005;96(9):1355–9. https://doi.org/10.1111/j.1464-410X.2005.05820.x.
75. Cao S, Yin X, Wang Y, Zhou H, Song F, Lu Z. Smoking and risk of erectile dysfunction: systematic review of observational studies with meta-analysis. PLoS One. 2013;8(4):e60443. https://doi.org/10.1371/journal.pone.0060443.
76. Harte CB, Meston CM. Association between smoking cessation and sexual health in men. BJU Int. 2012;109(6):888–96. https://doi.org/10.1111/j.1464-410X.2011.10503.x.
77. Pourmand G, Alidaee MR, Rasuli S, Maleki A, Mehrsai A. Do cigarette smokers with erectile dysfunction benefit from stopping?: a prospective study. BJU Int. 2004;94(9):1310–3. https://doi.org/10.1111/j.1464-410X.2004.05162.x.
78. Winter JE, MacInnis RJ, Wattanapenpaiboon N, Nowson CA. BMI and all-cause mortality in older adults: a meta-analysis. Am J Clin Nutr. 2014;99(4):875–90. https://doi.org/10.3945/ajcn.113.068122.
79. Porter Starr KN, Bales CW. Excessive body weight in older adults. Clin Geriatr Med. 2015;31(3):311–26. https://doi.org/10.1016/j.cger.2015.04.001.
80. Apostolopoulou M, Savopoulos C, Michalakis K, Coppack S, Dardavessis T, Hatzitolios A. Age, weight and obesity. Maturitas. 2012;71(2):115–9. https://doi.org/10.1016/j.maturitas.2011.11.015.
81. Smith L, Yang L, Forwood S, Lopez-Sanchez G, Koyanagi A, Veronese N, et al. Associations between sexual activity and weight status: findings from the English longitudinal study of ageing. PLoS One. 2019;14(9):e0221979. https://doi.org/10.1371/journal.pone.0221979.

82. Esposito K, Giugliano F, Ciotola M, De Sio M, D'Armiento M, Giugliano D. Obesity and sexual dysfunction, male and female. Int J Impot Res. 2008;20(4):358–65. https://doi.org/10.1038/ijir.2008.9.
83. Moon KH, Park SY, Kim YW. Obesity and erectile dysfunction: from bench to clinical implication. World J Mens Health. 2019;37(2):138–47. https://doi.org/10.5534/wjmh.180026.
84. Varghese M, Griffin C, McKernan K, Eter L, Abrishami S, Singer K. Female adipose tissue has improved adaptability and metabolic health compared to males in aged obesity. Aging. 2020;12(2):1725–46. https://doi.org/10.18632/aging.102709.
85. Esposito K, Giugliano D. Obesity, the metabolic syndrome, and sexual dysfunction in men. Clin Pharmacol Ther. 2011;90(1):169–73. https://doi.org/10.1038/clpt.2011.91.

Promotion of Sex in Older Adults

12

Hanna M. Mües, Kathrin Kirchheiner, and Igor Grabovac

By the year 2050, 22% of the world's population is expected to be aged 60 years and older [1]. The proportion of people over 60 years of age is therefore expected to nearly double from 900 million in 2015 (12% of the world's population) to a total of 2 billion in 2050. The so-called *population aging* was primarily observed in high-income countries and has now reached low- and middle-income countries as well and can hence be seen all around the world. For healthy individuals, more longevity can provide additional opportunities not only for one's own benefit but also for their family and society at large. In order to benefit from a longer life, however, physical and mental health are of utmost importance [1].

A central factor throughout human life that substantially contributes to health is sexuality [2]. Various studies have shown that sexual activity has a number of positive effects on the health and well-being of older adults. These include both physical (better cardiovascular health, improved immunity, lower incidence of some cancers) as well as mental health (lower depression, more satisfaction with mental health, greater quality of life). However, even though sexuality continues to be of importance in older adults, it is often underestimated in this age group. This is not only due to low research interest in this topic but also due to the surrounding social stigma that perpetuates the commonly adopted social image of a completely asexual

H. M. Mües (✉)
Department of Clinical and Health Psychology, Faculty of Psychology, University of Vienna, Vienna, Austria
e-mail: hanna.muees@univie.ac.at

K. Kirchheiner
Department of Radiation Oncology, Medical University of Vienna, Vienna, Austria
e-mail: kathrin.kirchheiner@akhwien.at

I. Grabovac
Department of Social and Preventive Medicine, Center for Public Health, Medical University of Vienna, Vienna, Austria
e-mail: igor.grabovac@meduniwien.ac.at

older person [3]. These issues may be even more prominent in older lesbian, gay, bisexual, transgender, intersex, and queer (LGBTIQ) people that often experience additional invisibility, given the usual societal perceptions of sexual orientation being connected with youth [4, 5]. These societal and cultural views perpetuate stereotypic views on sexuality and sex in older people, which further prevents research, education, and policies and in a way sustains the cycle of ill-information and misunderstanding.

There are particular challenges to sexuality and sexual health that are unique to aging adults [6]. Going into retirement, for example, might be accompanied by financial constraints and decreased healthcare access, which has a detrimental effect on the overall increased need for health care in older age. In addition, declines in physical and mental health can lead to an increasing need of support as well as a decrease in privacy either at home or in a retirement residency [6]. Living under such aggravated conditions can make it difficult for older adults to live out their sexuality freely and without constraints. Additionally, retirement, but also aging in general, is associated with a reduction in the size and quality of the social network which may further influence sexual activities and sexual health of older adults. In this context it is also important to note that losing one's partner is one of the most common factors associated with not reporting sexual activity in aging adults [7, 8].

In addition to the surrounding circumstances, aging involves physiological changes associated with drops in hormonal levels that may also affect sexual health. These include the decrease of estrogen, thinning and dryness of the vagina (atrophy of the vaginal mucosa), decreased vaginal lubrication, dyspareunia, and anorgasmia in women [6, 9, 10]. Aging-associated issues of sexual functioning in men include erectile dysfunction, decreased sexual desire, and anorgasmia. These issues are associated with a number of potential etiological factors [10, 11]. Overall, a certain degree of health is necessary to maintain sexual activity and as multimorbidity is also more prevalent in older adults, these also influence sexual health [12, 13]. For example, arthritis, rheumatism, and other health problems that limit mobility and cause pain may reduce sexual activity and show additional effects on mood and overall desire [14, 15]. Various chronic illnesses have been found associated with sexual dysfunction including obesity and diabetes, cardiac disease, prostate and ovarian cancer, stroke, renal disease, and lung disease [12, 13, 16, 17].

The advent of pharmaceuticals, marked by sildenafil citrate (Viagra) in 1998, and devices aiming for treatment of sexual dysfunction have been followed by constant and immense market growth, which further underlines the need for more attention of sexuality in older age by healthcare professionals and researchers [18]. Undoubtedly, these advances have provided much needed help to the people affected. However, they may have also increased unrealistic expectations of sexual functioning at almost any time and any age. These may lead to a vicious circle of added stress and pressure, increasing anxiety and creating additional problems causing further decline of sexual health and activity [19]. This anxiety may be amplified by assumptions of what is considered appropriate by society (also see Table 12.1) as well as assumptions that aging has negative effects on sexuality which, in women, could also decrease desire and increase the likelihood of non-pleasurable sex [10]. Moreover, female sexual

Table 12.1 Common sexual myths and misconceptions

1	Older adults do not engage in sex
2	Sex is best for younger adults
3	Individuals with disabilities, chronic pain, or in palliative care do not engage in sex
4	Only men are interested in sex and are always interested in and ready for sex
5	Sex is defined as penile-vaginal intercourse
6	Masturbation is not normal or continued in older age
7	Only gay men want anal sex
8	Orgasm is the only goal of sex
9	Satisfying the sexual partner does not need communication about sex
10	Risk of sexually transmitted infections and HIV among older populations is low

dysfunction is often related to their partner's desire. For example, some studies reported that when erectile function in male partners improved, so did sexual satisfaction and arousal in female partners [20]. These results are not to be generalized, and one should be aware that sexual desire is also closely related to emotional satisfaction, emotional closeness and intimacy as well as psychological factors. Given the myriad of positive aspects of sexuality in older adults as outlined in this book, it is necessary for healthcare workers to adequately address issues concerning sexuality when working with older adults. In particular, healthcare workers should be aware of challenges older adults face in the context of sexuality and consider the barriers when approaching these subjects working with this population.

12.1 Barriers to Communication on Sexual Health in Older Adults

There are a number of barriers in the form of sexual myths and misconceptions that prevent open and direct communication on sexual health with older adults as outlined in Table 12.1.

Older adults do not engage in sex. This and other sexual myths remain firm, but are false beliefs. Sexuality is often still treated as a taboo topic and not openly talked about. This is especially the case for older generations even though sexual satisfaction has been shown to be a predictor of life satisfaction in older adults [21]. Epidemiological research however shows that more than 80% of men and 65% of women aged 40–69 reported sexual intercourse in the past year [22]. Moreover, among studies on adults aged 85 to 95, one third reported sexual activities in the past year and 54% of men and women aged 75–85 reported having sex 2–3 times a month [3, 23]. Patients are often reluctant to start a conversation on sexuality, to ask any questions they might have on the topic or to talk about their sexual problems. Patients might feel ashamed of a lack of knowledge, including a lack of terminology, in this area or of any sexual problems they might have and might be afraid of being judged by the healthcare workers they confide in. Open communication about sexuality, however, is key to help correct wrong assumptions that might also prevent an individual from fully enjoying their sexuality. In a clinical context, the most common question asked by patients seems to be *"Is this normal?"* and the most common intervention therefore seems to be normalizing certain aspects of sexuality. Healthcare workers play a crucial role concerning the topic of sexuality and may serve as role models, as will be outlined further below.

Sex is best for younger adults. As has been stated above, various studies have shown a number of positive effects of sexual activity on the physical and mental health and well-being of older adults. Also, a 25-year follow-up study noted that frequency of sexual activity in men and enjoyment of sexual intercourse in women were associated with improved quality of life [24–31]. For more information, please see Chaps. 3–5.

Individuals with disabilities, chronic pain, or in palliative care do not engage in sex. Sexual needs and overall sexuality in people with disability, chronic pain, or those in palliative care are often overlooked, averted, or ignored by healthcare professionals as a vital part of holistic care. Data on these populations seems to be scarce, but the little research that is published shows that sexuality and intimacy remain important issues for a very large population [32–34]. For people with various degrees of disability, sexuality remains an important issue and is usually adapted by finding out the appropriate assistive devices or adequate positions. In chronic pain issues such as rheumatoid arthritis, studies reported between 31% and 76% of sexual dysfunction, which was also most associated with pain, joint stiffness, and fatigue [35]. Synthetized data from 44,750 participants showed a 1.7-fold and a 1.9-fold increased risk of sexual dysfunction in men and women with rheumatoid arthritis, respectively [36]. Similar results are seen in patients with chronic lower back pain. For patients receiving palliative care, there are some indices of high prevalence of sexual dysfunction in the palliative care population. Moreover, the prevalence also seems to vary among different underlying illnesses; for example 52% of patients with advanced cancer reported no sexual intercourse and only 12% described sexual satisfaction as "good" [34]. According to a study by Kelemen et al. [37], almost 92% of palliative care patients reported never having been asked about sexuality and intimacy but 48% considered that their illness significantly impacted intimacy in a negative way. This is concerning as 86% of patients at a palliative care unit claimed this topic to be important enough to want to talk to a knowledgeable expert about it [34]. Most authors conclude that sexual counseling and open dialogue with healthcare professionals are key. As part of a routine first assessment questionnaire, questions on intimacy and privacy with the partner could be included and updated regularly. Furthermore, handing out room keys or "do not disturb" signs for single rooms or, if single rooms are not available, offering an extra room could provide opportunities for patient privacy.

Only men are interested in sex and are always interested in and ready for sex. Many men experience a lack of sexual desire that may be associated with a lack of testicular function and low testosterone levels. On the whole, lower sexual drive or desire may be caused by a variety of endocrine, organic, or psychological factors that may be more closely related to declining overall health rather than aging itself [38]. However, lower sex drive might result in relational distress due to the cultural expectations of men as always being interested in or ready for sex. It should be added that many men do retain interest in sex even if their desire is lower and that sexuality also remains important to many women in later life [32, 39].

Sex is defined as penile-vaginal intercourse. Sexuality is broad and sexual activities may be defined in various ways, with most research on older adults usually focusing on a variety of activities. This is usually necessary as penile-vaginal sex activities decline in frequency with physiological changes. In addition to penile-vaginal sex, studies that describe sexual activities include displays of affection such as kissing, masturbation, petting, fondling, oral sex, and anal sex [29, 40]. However, studies report that more than 80% of men and women over the age of 65 report regular penile-vaginal intercourse [41]. Such results should be interpreted with caution given the high variability among different geographical areas and study methods [42].

Masturbation is not normal or continued in older age. A cross-sectional international study found that in adults aged 60–75 years most masturbation was reported among Norwegian men (65%) and women (40%), while the lowest was found in Portugal with 42% and 27% in the past month (where most intercourse was reported) [42]. A Scottish study of a convenience sample showed that 15% of people older than 65 reported engaging in masturbation in the past month but also only 2% of participants said that this activity was important or very important [29].

Only gay men want anal sex. In general, data on nonpenetrative sexual activities and non-vaginal intercourse is very rare and almost nonexistent in older adults. Anal sexual activity in heterosexual adults in general is not rare, and the overall lifetime prevalence (i.e., the proportion of individuals who report anal sexual activity at some point in their life) reported in an extensive systematic review was 22%. Furthermore, the authors stated that in studies on frequencies of different sexual activities including anal sexual activity, between 3% and 24% of all sexual activities reported were anal intercourse, with great differences among studies and methodologies used [43].

Orgasm is the only goal of sex. There are several reasons for engaging in sexual activities, including but not limited to orgasms. Meston and Buss [44] found the following four main factors for undergraduate students to engage in sexual intercourse: physical reasons, goal attainment reasons, emotional reasons, and insecurity reasons. Out of 237 most frequently named items, women ranked the achievement of an orgasm as the 14th and men as the ninth most important reason to engage in sexual intercourse [44]. In another study, Mark et al. [45] found that men were more likely to desire orgasm, sexual release, and to please the partner, while women were more likely to want intimacy, emotional closeness, love, and to feel desirable [45]. In a study by Kalra et al. [46], 83% of adults aged 60 years and older reported worse orgasms than when they were at a younger age. At the same time, a reported decrease in orgasm intensity, which was higher in individuals with illness, did not distress 71.4% of individuals. Healthy and working individuals adjusted best and expected age-related orgasmic change [46]. Other studies however found that the ability to reach orgasm remains important to older adults, especially to men [47]. Nevertheless, it has also been reported by men that the focus of experiencing sexuality in older age shifts from intercourse to touch, sensuality, and intimacy, thereby opening up new possibilities [48].

Satisfying the sexual partner does not need communication about sex. Sexual communication has been repeatedly shown to be associated with both higher relationship satisfaction and sexual satisfaction [49, 50]. In older adults open communication about sex, including talking about and seeking help for sexual issues, can enhance an active and satisfying sexual life [51]. Sexual communication therefore keeps playing an important role for this age group.

Risk of sexually transmitted infections and HIV among older populations is low. Contrasting the myth of the asexual older adult, sexually transmitted infections (STIs) such as primary and secondary syphilis (2008: 0.8 cases per 100,000; 2018: 2.5 cases per 100,000), early latent syphilis (2008: 0.8 cases per 100,000; 2018: 3.0 cases per 100,000), chlamydia (2008: 5.5 cases per 100,000; 2018: 16 cases per 100,000), and gonorrhea (2008: 4.5 cases per 100,000; 2018: 15.5 cases per 100,000) have increased among adults over 55 years of age in the USA [52]. While HIV prevalence (2008: 173.9 cases per 100,000; 2018: 380.4 cases per 100,000) has also increased in this age group, HIV diagnoses have decreased (2008: 5.7 cases per 100,000; 2018: 4.0 cases per 100,000) [52]. Risk factors may include age-related physiological changes, psychosocial changes such as loss of partner, and risky sexual behavior [53]. However, opportunities to test for HIV and STIs, which could help prevent further spreading and increase quality of lives, seem to be missed [54]. Sexual history taking, which could help to identify individuals at risk, is not carried out frequently even though most older adults would be open to discussing sexual health with their healthcare professional, and many preferring their healthcare professional to take the initiative [54].

Healthcare workers play an essential role in creating the necessary conditions for older adults to entrust themselves and to enable open communication about their sexuality. However, general practitioners often do not seem to proactively discuss sexual health with older patients [55]. One issue is time availability for such a careful discussion in a busy clinical routine. Furthermore, talking about sexuality is sometimes perceived as inappropriate and potentially harmful to the doctor-patient relationship, and related issues such as STI prevention are not viewed as relevant to this population. In addition, many general practitioners feel uncomfortable discussing sexual health with this age group and have little knowledge and training on this [55].

12.2 Healthcare Worker's Knowledge on and Experience with Sexuality in Older Adults

An important aspect of the *Sexual Rights* is the right to "*the highest attainable standard of sexual health, including access to sexual and reproductive health care services*" ([2], p. 5). A prerequisite to fulfill this right is appointing healthcare workers with sufficient knowledge of the subject and of appropriate treatment and care, and who have the ability and willingness to share and discuss sexuality-related information appropriately and comfortably [2]. However, healthcare workers often do not have the necessary education on sexuality in older adults, assuming their asexuality and low risk of sexually transmitted infections [6]. Furthermore, sexual health issues are often addressed with an "easy and quick fix", such as a prescription. While this may solve some, but not all problems for male patients, there is a lack of such options for female patients. This may lead to the false assumption that other sexual problems cannot be treated in older adults and instead have to be accepted as a part of aging even though, with special training, evidence-based interventions are available.

Sexual health as an important part of everyday functioning and quality of life should also be one of the tenets of a holistic approach to patient health. This means that questions of sexual health (treatment of dysfunction as well as promotion of sexual health) should be viewed from a multidisciplinary angle, with various experts from health and health allied fields such as medical doctors, psychologists, psychotherapists, occupational therapists, nurses, and pharmacists being consulted. A general issue is the overall lack of training among health and allied health professionals, which is also reflected in the paucity of studies dealing with knowledge and attitudes of healthcare workers on sex and sexuality. A Turkish-based study reported limited knowledge and information on sexuality in older adults by medical doctors, while a study of nurses in Flemish homes for the elderly showed rather positive attitudes towards sexuality in older people and moderate levels of knowledge [56, 57].

12.2.1 Education of Healthcare Professionals in the Context of Sexuality

Education of professionals relevant to the healthcare system should include several aspects in the context of sexuality. Knowledge of the term sexuality is required, which includes "sex, gender identities and roles, sexual orientation, eroticism, pleasure, intimacy and reproduction. Sexuality is experienced and expressed in thoughts, fantasies, desires, beliefs, attitudes, values, behaviors, practices, roles and relationships. While sexuality can include all of these dimensions, not all of them are always experienced or expressed. Sexuality is influenced by the interaction of biological, psychological, social, economic, political, cultural, ethical, legal, historical, religious and spiritual factors" ([2], p. 5). A basic knowledge of sex organs, sexual feelings, sexual activities and sexual problems as well as language and terminology should therefore be acquired to enable healthcare workers to talk openly and easily [58].

Furthermore, depending on the profession, techniques, tools, treatment options, and evidence-based sexual health interventions should be taught as part of healthcare worker's training [58]. For example, an exploration of the patient's sexual history should be a natural part of a careful anamnesis (for more details see *3. Discussing sexuality-related topics in a professional context*). Education on sexuality should also take into account the background and characteristics of patients, including their age, which also become apparent during the anamnesis.

In addition to knowledge and practical tools on the topic, healthcare workers who personally feel comfortable with the topic of sexuality show congruence between nonverbal and verbal communication in contrast to incongruence which hinders support (for more details see *3. Discussing sexuality-related topics in a professional context*). The role sexuality plays in the healthcare worker's life could be explored in order to experience it as an enriching part of life and to take on a reflective attitude. For example, for psychotherapists in training this could be done as part of their encounter groups [58]. Medical doctors might be able to use Balint groups as an opportunity to discuss and reflect on this topic [59]. These and similar possibilities could help healthcare workers to feel more comfortable with this topic.

12.2.2 Evaluation of Sexual Health Services

A more detailed evaluation of factors that are important in the context of sexuality for healthcare workers working with older adults is shown in Table 12.2. Based on the WHO's *Guiding principles for successful programme interventions in sexual health (2006, p. 20)*, Barrett [60] suggested 17 dichotomous statements that can be used to evaluate sexual health services for older adults. The authors of this chapter adapted and extended Barrett's statements to 23 statements. A high total number of statements answered with "yes" indicate greater compliance with the WHO principles [60]. The statements relate to the following themes: healthcare workers' knowledge and willingness, the right to sexual health, affirmative approach and autonomy, comprehensive understanding, cultural diversity, equity, addressing sexual violence and abuse, privacy and confidentiality, non-judgmental services, and accountability and responsibility.

Table 12.2 Evaluation of sexual health services and healthcare workers (HCWs) for older adults. An adaptation and extension of Barrett ([60], p. 36) based on WHO [2]

		Response	
Item	Statement	Yes	No
	Instruction: Please tick yes or no to each statement		
1	Strategies promoting sexual health are in accordance with evidence-based and up to date practice.		
2	HCWs have sufficient knowledge of the subject and of appropriate treatment and care [2].		
3	HCWs have the ability and willingness to discuss sexuality-related information appropriately and comfortably [2]. HCWs recognize all rights of others, including the *Sexual Rights* ([2], p.5), and as such, among others, recognize the rights of older adults to: 　(a) The highest attainable sexual health standard and access to sexual and reproductive healthcare services and education on sexuality. 　(b) Bodily integrity#[2]. 　(c) Choose their partner(s). 　(d) Decide to be sexually active or not. 　(e) Consensual sexual life and marriage#[2]. 　(f) A satisfying, safe, and pleasurable sex life.		
4	HCWs take an open-minded and positive approach to sexual health and sexual expression, and address pleasure and safety.		
5	HCWs recognize their patient's right to make free and informed decisions about their lives, including their sexuality.		
6	HCWs understand the biopsychosocial changes that occur in the course of a life span, incorporate their knowledge into their work, and, if appropriate, share it with older adults.		
7	HCWs understand that information patients share on their sexuality is private and sensitive information that patients share solely voluntarily and for which confidentiality rules apply.		
8	HCWs advocate for and actively engage in sexual health promotion.		
9	HCWs take into account their patient's factors such as sexual orientation, illness, culture, age, and disability#[2].		
10	HCWs are supported to self-reflect on their own culture, values, and beliefs and their possible impact on patient care.		
11	Procedures for sexual health promotion actively consider the inclusivity of gay, lesbian, bisexual, trans, and intersex people.		
12	Cultural sensitivity actively accounts for gender imbalances and stereotypes in provision of services that focuses on the needs specific to male, female and transgender older people.		
13	HCWs are acutely aware of potential sexual abuse issues of older adults including unwanted sexual acts, sexual contact, rape, language, or other exploitative behavior where the consent was not given or was obtained through coercion.		
14	HCWs understand their duties and responsibilities when it comes to mandatory reporting of sexual abuse and their role in the prevention of sexually abusive behaviors.		
15	HCWs respect their patients' preferences, views, and values without judging them or forcing their own views upon them.		
16	HCWs understand the importance of accessibility, affordability, confidentiality, high-quality, and age- and culture-appropriateness of sexual health programs#[2].		
17	Health care services ensure the compliance with the abovementioned principles through continuous monitoring and iterative processes that maintain the quality of services for promotion of sexual health of older people.		

12.3 Discussing Sexuality-Related Topics in a Professional Context

Enquiring about a patient's sexual health should be self-evident as it is an important aspect of health. However, the topic is often neglected by healthcare workers. Approaching the topic of sexuality in older people requires an understanding of the barriers that have been discussed above as well as sufficient knowledge and the ability and willingness to talk about sexuality appropriately und comfortably [2]. Before starting a conversation on sexuality in a professional context, a few basic rules of communication need to be pointed out.

12.3.1 Basic Rules of Communication

While the content of a conversation is of importance, nonverbal communication also plays a critical role to establish trust as well as a successful patient-healthcare worker relationship. As the first of five axioms of communication by Watzlawick et al. [61] states, it is not possible to not communicate. Healthcare workers should therefore be aware of their body language, speaking speed, tone of voice, use of pauses, and other forms of nonverbal communication as they influence a conversation. Furthermore, as the second axiom states, communication has a content aspect as well as a relationship aspect, and the relationship aspect determines the content [61]. The content aspect will be discussed further later. The role of a good relationship between healthcare workers and their patients should not be underestimated. In the case of psychotherapists for example, the patient-therapist relationship explains 30% of the variance in patient outcome and is therefore the most significant factor of therapist activities to contribute to therapy outcome [62]. According to the fifth axiom by Watzlawick et al. [61] there are two different kinds of relationships: a symmetric and a complementary one. While symmetric relationships are based on the equality of the individuals involved, complementary relationships are based on differences due to the fact that one person has a superior position to the other [61]. The patient-healthcare worker relationship classifies as the latter, as for example, the healthcare worker knows much more about the patient than does the patient of the healthcare worker. Healthcare workers should be aware of the inequality of their relationship and handle it responsibly.

According to Carl Rogers [63], congruence, acceptance, and empathy provided by the therapist are necessary conditions for a successful relationship between a client and a therapist. According to Rogers, a therapist shows congruence, genuineness, and integration if "within the relationship he is freely and deeply himself, with his actual experience accurately represented by his awareness of himself. It is the opposite of presenting a facade, either knowingly or unknowingly" ([63], p. 97). Authenticity is an important key term. The aim is to be aware of one's own feelings, while not necessarily sharing them with the patient, and not to deceive the patient as to one's self. It means to be a real and genuine person, consistent in verbal and nonverbal communication, without presenting an empty professional role but being based on values and ethics. By acceptance, the next condition, Rogers describes unconditional positive regard "of each aspect of the client's experience as being a part of that client" ([63], p. 98). Furthermore, "it means a caring for the client as a *separate* person, with permission to have his own feelings, his own experiences" ([63], p. 98). The patient is therefore met without judgment of aspects of the patient being "good" or "bad". It is possible to disagree with or even reject certain behaviors of the patient, while still fully accepting the person itself. The third condition, empathy, means "experiencing an accurate, empathic understanding of the client's awareness of his own experience. To sense the client's private world as if it were your own, but without ever losing the 'as if' quality" ([63], p. 99). It describes shifting the perspective and seeing the world through the patient's eyes or walking a mile in their shoes without losing one's own self in the process and with the ability to switch back at any time. These three factors, congruence, acceptance, and empathy, can also be helpful for a conversation between a healthcare worker and a patient. Further useful conversational skills are provided by the technique of active listening, which goes back to Rogers and Farson [64], as it demonstrates empathy, respect, and understanding. It requires the listener to listen from the patient's point of view and to convey this to him or her. The active listener is attentive of the total meaning of the message including underlying feelings, and notes nonverbal cues, as has been described earlier [64]. Picking up emotional cues in patients and mirroring them through facial expressions may lead to the patient seeing their own grief in the active listener's face, which may increase the feeling of being understood. Furthermore, the active listener reacts nonverbally with behaviors including nods, eye contact, and a facing posture, and verbally including paraphrasing, verbalizing feelings, and asking questions [65]. The verbal reactions will be described further in the following sentences. Paraphrasing, which means repeating or describing what the patient has communicated using one's own words, can be used to ensure true understanding of the patient and to avoid misunderstandings. Verbalizing feelings, which means reflecting on the conveyed feelings of the patient and verbalizing them carefully, may allow patients to be more aware of their feelings, and carefully offering them an interpretation may help patients to reach a higher level of awareness. However, it is important to keep in mind that the patient is the expert of his or her feelings and that the listener should, if uncertain, rather ask the patient how he or she felt about something. Fast interpretations or insensitive confrontations should be avoided [65]. When asking questions, the following hints should be considered. First, open questions are preferred to closed questions as they invite the patient to open up and give more elaborate answers instead of short, desirable (in the case of leading questions) or simple yes/no answers. Furthermore, questions starting with "why…?" might imply criticism and judgment and should therefore be avoided. At the beginning of a conversation, it is recommended to start with general questions and questions about facts and to later go on to more specific and personal questions [66].

During the conversation, pauses might occur which can have different causes. When a pause occurs, it is advised to consider the cause of the pause and the previous content of the conversation to, if necessary, be able to help the patient to continue, rather than to think about the pause itself. The patient might want a pause to think, e.g., about how much to open up to the healthcare worker or to try to find the right words, in which case it is suggested to wait patiently, while staying in an active listening pose. A pause might also indicate that the patient has trouble remembering or it might have emotional causes. If the patient seems to look for help or avoids eye contact, it can be appropriate for healthcare workers to offer help to the patient by, e.g., repeating or summarizing parts of the previous conversation, by telling the patient to take their time, or by verbalizing that it seems to be hard for the patient to talk about the topic. It can also be appropriate not to continue with a topic that, e.g., is stressful for the patient to talk about and therefore to offer this option to the patient [66].

As has been noted previously, the second axiom by Watzlawick et al. states that communication has a content aspect as well as a relationship aspect, and the relationship aspect determines the content [61]. Since the relationship aspect has already been discussed, the content aspect will now be focused on further using the communication square by Schulz von Thun [67]. The communication square postulates that a message that is sent by a sender and received by a receiver has four facets which might be perceived with different emphasis. The four facets are factual information, self-revelation, relationship, and appeal. The factual information includes the objective information stated in the message (which information is given?). Self-revelation describes the information that a message (willingly or unwillingly) provides on its sender (what does the message show about the sender?). The relationship facet gives information on the sender's thoughts and feelings towards the receiver and the relationship between sender and receiver (what information is given on the receiver and the relationship between the sender and receiver?). The appeal describes what the sender intends to achieve regarding the receiver (e.g., advice; what does the sender want from the receiver or what does the sender expect the receiver to do?). As a receiver, the aim is to be aware of all four facets of a message and to consciously decide on the reaction to the message, depending on the situation [67].

In summary, healthcare workers are advised to be aware of their verbal as well as their nonverbal communication. Furthermore, they should keep the content aspect as well as the relationship aspect of communication in mind and be aware of their complementary, not symmetric, relationship to their patients and the possibly beneficial effect of congruence, acceptance, and empathy on their relationships with their patients. Techniques of active listening and awareness of pauses as well as of the four facets of a message may be of further use for healthcare workers.

12.3.2 Initiating a Conversation on Sexuality

Now that some basic communication rules have been established, the question of how to initiate a conversation on sexuality rises. Patients themselves are often ashamed or afraid of bringing up this topic. It is therefore helpful to provide opportunities for patients while keeping them comfortable and at ease. Possible approaches strongly depend on the professional background of the healthcare professional and the circumstances. In a general setting, such as general practitioner consultation without any obvious relation to sexuality, the topic could be introduced as follows: "In medicine, we regard sexual health as an important part of physical health and general quality of life. Would you be comfortable if we address some questions?" If possible, sexual health can be assessed after establishing a solid rapport with the patient rather than at the first consultation. In a gynecologic-oncologic setting with obvious relation to sexuality, the conversation is more straightforward as treatment might cause damage to the vagina, which might lead to sexual dysfunctions. In this context, patients also receive information about vaginal changes after treatment and are taught basic interventions to prevent consequential problems.

The patient is thereby free to choose whether he or she wants to talk about their sexuality or decline the invitation politely by not going into the topic. Depending on the healthcare worker's profession and the importance of the issue with a particular patient, healthcare workers can emphasize the importance of discussing sexual health as part of, for example, a medical examination.

When a patient chooses to talk about their sexuality or sexual problems, healthcare workers are advised to listen carefully, keep an open mind, and be empathic. Depending on their training and qualification, they might ask further questions, suggest an appropriate treatment, and answer any questions that come up. They could also suggest a contact point at which the patient can find answers and help.

12.3.3 Exploring Sexual History

As mentioned above, exploring the sexual history should be a natural part of an anamnesis. The following guide is based on the Guide to Taking a Sexual History [68] as well as experiences of the authors. It should be taken as a framework that needs to be adapted to the specific cultural setting and amended according to individual patients. Some patients may not feel comfortable to talk about sexuality or sexual activities and it should be clearly stated that this is a normal part of their exam and important for their health.

1. Please outline your intentions clearly: "I will ask you some questions about sexual activities and your sexual health. These may be very personal and private, but they are important for your overall health and well-being. I ask these questions to all my adult patients regardless of their age, gender identity, sexual orientation, or marital status. Please be assured that everything discussed is treated with strict confidentiality".
2. Never assume the sexual orientation or gender identity of your patient. When asking questions on the number of sexual partners, keep in mind that if only one partner is noted in the past year, ask about potential risk behavior of the partner (length of the relationship, current or past sexual partners, drug use). If more partners are noted, explore individual risk factors additionally (such as condom use). Some questions examples: "Are you currently sexually active?", "Do you share intimacy with another person?", "Do you integrate sexual self-care in your

private life? (Are you sexually active with yourself?)", "Are you currently in an exclusive relationship (monogamy) or any other kind of relationship that is more loose?", "In recent months how many sexual partners have you had?", "What genders were the sexual partners?".

If the patient states no partners skip the next step.

3. If the patient reported more than one sexual partner in the past year, you should explore the sexual practices in more detail. These are important to assess risk and also to guide further steps you may need to take (such as sample collection). Keep in mind that in assessing sexual activities in older adults, questions regarding nonpenetrative sexual activities may be especially important. Again, ask questions clearly: "Now I may be a bit more explicit with you, asking you about the kind of sex you had in the past 12 months. Please keep in mind that sexual activity is not exclusively defined as intercourse. What kind of sexual activities have you had?". If necessary, you should clearly ask about specific sexual activities: "Have you engaged in any…" (a) "kissing?", (b) "cuddling?", (c) "caressing?", (d) "petting?", (e) "mutual masturbation?", (f) "manual, oral or sex toy stimulation?", (g) "vaginal intercourse?", (h) "anal sex?", or (i) "other activities?".

4. Be sure to assess signs or symptoms of sexual problems or dysfunctions. Again, try to ask open questions, when possible and be more specific, if necessary. "Have you noticed any difficulties when having sex (with yourself or with your partner(s))?", "Have you noticed any problems with your libido/a lack of sexual desire or the inability to initiate sexual activities that bother you?", "Are there any problems with your reactions of arousal that bother you (erectile functioning or lack of lubrication)?", "Are there any changes in reaching an orgasm that bother you?", "Have you experienced any discomfort or pain during sex?", "Have you experienced any mental or psychological distress during sexual activities?" If you identify any potential issues and problems, please continue with a more detailed clinical examination and history to create a working differential diagnosis and plan a diagnostic and treatment plan.

5. When it comes to protection used, be aware that older adults may be less informed about the need for safe sex and you should individually assess the level of risk. It is important not only to assess the risk but also the patient's own perceptions of risk. This step is also an important step in risk reduction and prevention and advice on safe sex practices should be given and reinforced in all patients. Examples "How would you estimate your personal risk for sexually transmitted diseases?", "Have you used any protection when having sex? If not, could you tell me the reason? If yes, what sort of protection have you used?" "How often do you use this type of protection?" If not always: "Could you tell me about some situation when you did not use protection and with whom?". Be sure to assess the history of sexually transmitted diseases: "Have you ever been diagnosed with a sexually transmitted disease?", "Have you had any recurring symptoms?", "Have you ever been tested for an STD?", "Would you like to be tested today?".

6. Be sure to allow enough time for patients to ask you additional questions and directly ask: "Do you have any questions for me?", "Is there anything else you would like to discuss with me today?".

References

1. World Health Organization. Aging and health. 2018. https://www.who.int/news-room/fact-sheets/detail/ageing-and-health#:~:text=By%202050%2C%20the%20world's%20population,in%20this%20age%20group%20worldwide.
2. World Health Organization. Defining sexual health: report of a technical consultation of sexual health, 28–31 January 2002. Geneva: Sexual health document series; 2006. http://www.who.int/reproductivehealth/publications/sexual_health/defining_sexual_health.pdf.
3. Hyde Z, Flicker L, Hankey GJ, Almeida OP, McCaul KA, Chubb SA, Yeap BB. Prevalence of sexual activity and associated factors in men aged 75 to 95 years: a cohort study. Ann Intern Med. 2010;153(11):693–702. https://doi.org/10.7326/0003-4819-153-11-201012070-00002.
4. Grabovac I, Smith L, McDermott DT, Stefanac S, Yang L, Veronese N, Jackson SE. Well-being among older gay and bisexual men and women in England: a cross-sectional population study. J Am Med Dir Assoc. 2019;20(9):1080–1085.e1081. https://doi.org/10.1016/j.jamda.2019.01.119.
5. Knochel KA, Croghan CF, Moone RP, Quam JK. Training, geography, and provision of aging services to lesbian, gay, bisexual, and transgender older adults. J Gerontol Soc Work. 2012;55(5):426–43. https://doi.org/10.1080/01634372.2012.665158.
6. World Health Organization. WHO meeting on ethical, legal, human rights and social accountability implications of self-care interventions for sexual and reproductive health: 12–14 March 2018, Brocher Foundation, Hermance, Switzerland: summary report. Geneva: World Health Organization; 2018.
7. Matthias RE, Lubben JE, Atchison KA, Schweitzer SO. Sexual activity and satisfaction among very old adults: results from a community-dwelling Medicare population survey. Gerontologist. 1997;37(1):6–14. https://doi.org/10.1093/geront/37.1.6.
8. Smith LJ, Mulhall JP, Deveci S, Monaghan N, Reid MC. Sex after seventy: a pilot study of sexual function in older persons. J Sex Med. 2007;4(5):1247–53. https://doi.org/10.1111/j.1743-6109.2007.00568.x.
9. Ambler DR, Bieber EJ, Diamond MP. Sexual function in elderly women: a review of current literature. Rev Obstet Gynecol. 2012;5(1):16–27. https://www.ncbi.nlm.nih.gov/pubmed/22582123.
10. Laumann EO, Nicolosi A, Glasser DB, Paik A, Gingell C, Moreira E, Wang T. Sexual problems among women and men aged 40–80y: prevalence and correlates identified in the global study of sexual attitudes and behaviors. Int J Impot Res. 2005;17:39–57. https://doi.org/10.1038/sj.ijir.3901250.
11. Mulhall JP, Luo X, Zou KH, Stecher V, Galaznik A. Relationship between age and erectile dysfunction diagnosis or treatment using real-world observational data in the USA. Int J Clin Pract. 2016;70(12):1012–8. https://doi.org/10.1111/ijcp.12908.
12. Camacho ME, Reyes-Ortiz CA. Sexual dysfunction in the elderly: age or disease? Int J Impot Res. 2005;17:S52–6. https://doi.org/10.1038/sj.ijir.3901429.
13. Ni Lochlainn M, Kenny RA. Sexual activity and aging. J Am Med Dir Assoc. 2013;14(8):565–72. https://doi.org/10.1016/j.jamda.2013.01.022.
14. Dorner TE, Berner C, Haider S, Grabovac I, Lamprecht T, Fenzl KH, Erlacher L. Sexual health in patients with rheumatoid arthritis and the association between physical fitness and sexual function: a cross-sectional study. Rheumatol Int. 2018;38(6):1103–14. https://doi.org/10.1007/s00296-018-4023-3.

15. Grabovac I, Dorner TE. Association between low back pain and various everyday performances: activities of daily living, ability to work and sexual function. Wien Klin Wochenschr. 2019;131(21–22):541–9. https://doi.org/10.1007/s00508-019-01542-7.
16. Maiorino MI, Bellastella G, Esposito K. Diabetes and sexual dysfunction: current perspectives. Diabetes Metab Syndr Obes. 2014;7:95–105. https://doi.org/10.2147/DMSO.S36455.
17. Palacios S, Castaño R, Grazziotin A. Epidemiology of female sexual dysfunction. Maturitas. 2009;63(2):119–23. https://doi.org/10.1016/j.maturitas.2009.04.002.
18. Tiefer L. Medicalizations and demedicalizations of sexuality therapies. J Sex Res. 2012;49(4):311–8. https://doi.org/10.1080/00224499.2012.678948.
19. Marshall BL. Medicalization and the refashioning of age-related limits on sexuality. J Sex Res. 2012;49(4):337–43. https://doi.org/10.1080/00224499.2011.644597.
20. Goldstein I, Fisher WA, Sand M, Rosen RC, Mollen M, Brock G, et al. Women's sexual function improves when partners are administered vardenafil for erectile dysfunction: a prospective, randomized, double-blind, placebo-controlled trial. J Sex Med. 2005;2(6):819–32. https://doi.org/10.1111/j.1743-6109.2005.00147.x.
21. Skałacka K, Gerymski R. Sexual activity and life satisfaction in older adults. Psychogeriatrics. 2019;19(3):195–201. https://doi.org/10.1111/psyg.12381.
22. Nicolosi A, Laumann EO, Glasser DB, Moreira ED, Paik A, Gingell C, Global Study of Sexual Attitudes and Behaviors Investigators' Group. Sexual behavior and sexual dysfunctions after age 40: the global study of sexual attitudes and behaviors. Urology. 2004;64(5):991–7. https://doi.org/10.1016/j.urology.2004.06.055.
23. Lindau ST, Gavrilova N. Sex, health, and years of sexually active life gained due to good health: evidence from two US population based cross sectional surveys of ageing. BMJ. 2010;340:c810. https://doi.org/10.1136/bmj.c810.
24. Bosland MC. The etiopathogenesis of prostatic cancer with special reference to environmental factors. Adv Cancer Res. 1988;51:1–106. https://doi.org/10.1016/s0065-230x(08)60220-1.
25. Brody S. The relative health benefits of different sexual activities. J Sex Med. 2010;7(4 Pt 1):1336–61. https://doi.org/10.1111/j.1743-6109.2009.01677.x.
26. Brody S, Costa RM. Satisfaction (sexual, life, relationship, and mental health) is associated directly with penile-vaginal intercourse, but inversely with other sexual behavior frequencies. J Sex Med. 2009;6(7):1947–54. https://doi.org/10.1111/j.1743-6109.2009.01303.x.
27. Brody S, Preut R. Vaginal intercourse frequency and heart rate variability. J Sex Marital Ther. 2003;29(5):371–80. https://doi.org/10.1080/00926230390224747.
28. Ebrahim S, May M, Ben Shlomo Y, McCarron P, Frankel S, Yarnell J, Davey Smith G. Sexual intercourse and risk of ischaemic stroke and coronary heart disease: the Caerphilly study. J Epidemiol Community Health. 2002;56(2):99–102. https://doi.org/10.1136/jech.56.2.99.
29. Flynn TJ, Gow AJ. Examining associations between sexual behaviours and quality of life in older adults. Age Ageing. 2015;44(5):823–8. https://doi.org/10.1093/ageing/afv083.
30. Lê MG, Bachelot A, Hill C. Characteristics of reproductive life and risk of breast cancer in a case-control study of young nulliparous women. J Clin Epidemiol. 1989;42(12):1227–33. https://doi.org/10.1016/0895-4356(89)90121-2.
31. Palmore EB. Predictors of the longevity difference: a 25-year follow-up. Gerontologist. 1982;22(6):513–8. https://doi.org/10.1093/geront/22.6.513.
32. Lemieux L, Kaiser S, Pereira J, Meadows LM. Sexuality in palliative care: patient perspectives. Palliat Med. 2004;18(7):630–7. https://doi.org/10.1191/0269216304pm941oa.
33. Rouanne M, Massard C, Hollebecque A, Rousseau V, Varga A, Gazzah A, et al. Evaluation of sexuality, health-related quality-of-life and depression in advanced cancer patients: a prospective study in a phase I clinical trial unit of predominantly targeted anticancer drugs. Eur J Cancer. 2013;49(2):431–8. https://doi.org/10.1016/j.ejca.2012.08.008.
34. Vitrano V, Catania V, Mercadante S. Sexuality in patients with advanced cancer: a prospective study in a population admitted to an acute pain relief and palliative care unit. Am J Hosp Palliat Med. 2011;28(3):198–202. https://doi.org/10.1177/1049909110386044.
35. Tristano AG. Impact of rheumatoid arthritis on sexual function. World J Orthop. 2014;5(2):107–11. https://doi.org/10.5312/wjo.v5.i2.107.

36. Zhao S, Li E, Wang J, Luo L, Luo J, Zhao Z. Rheumatoid arthritis and risk of sexual dysfunction: a systematic review and Metaanalysis. J Rheumatol. 2018;45(10):1375–82. https://doi.org/10.3899/jrheum.170956.
37. Kelemen A, Cagle J, Chung J, Groninger H. Assessing the impact of serious illness on patient intimacy and sexuality in palliative care. J Pain Symptom Manag. 2019;58(2):282–8. https://doi.org/10.1016/j.jpainsymman.2019.04.015.
38. Chung E. Sexuality in ageing male: review of pathophysiology and treatment strategies for various male sexual dysfunctions. Med Sci (Basel). 2019;7(10):98. https://doi.org/10.3390/medsci7100098.
39. Moreira ED, Glasser DB, Gingell C, GSSAB Investigators' Group. Sexual activity, sexual dysfunction and associated help-seeking behaviours in middle-aged and older adults in Spain: a population survey. World J Urol. 2005;23(6):422–9. https://doi.org/10.1007/s00345-005-0035-1.
40. Smith L, Yang L, Forwood S, Lopez-Sanchez G, Koyanagi A, Veronese N, et al. Associations between sexual activity and weight status: findings from the English longitudinal study of ageing. PLoS One. 2019;14(9):e0221979. https://doi.org/10.1371/journal.pone.0221979.
41. Lindau ST, Schumm LP, Laumann EO, Levinson W, O'Muircheartaigh CA, Waite LJ. A study of sexuality and health among older adults in the United States. N Engl J Med. 2007;357(8):762–74. https://doi.org/10.1056/NEJMoa067423.
42. Træen B, Štulhofer A, Janssen E, Carvalheira AA, Hald GM, Lange T, Graham C. Sexual activity and sexual satisfaction among older adults in four European countries. Arch Sex Behav. 2019;48(3):815–29. https://doi.org/10.1007/s10508-018-1256-x.
43. Owen BN, Brock PM, Butler AR, Pickles M, Brisson M, Baggaley RF, Boily MC. Prevalence and frequency of heterosexual anal intercourse among young people: a systematic review and meta-analysis. AIDS Behav. 2015;19(7):1338–60. https://doi.org/10.1007/s10461-015-0997-y.
44. Meston CM, Buss DM. Why humans have sex. Arch Sex Behav. 2007;36(4):477–507. https://doi.org/10.1007/s10508-007-9175-2.
45. Mark K, Herbenick D, Fortenberry D, Sanders S, Reece M. The object of sexual desire: examining the "what" in "what do you desire?". J Sex Med. 2014;11(11):2709–19. https://doi.org/10.1111/jsm.12683.
46. Kalra G, Subramanyam A, Pinto C. Sexuality: desire, activity and intimacy in the elderly. Indian J Psychiatry. 2011;53(4):300–6. https://doi.org/10.4103/0019-5545.91902.
47. Helgason AR, Adolfsson J, Dickman P, Arver S, Fredrikson M, Göthberg M, Steineck G. Sexual desire, erection, orgasm and ejaculatory functions and their importance to elderly Swedish men: a population-based study. Age Ageing. 1996;25(4):285–91. https://doi.org/10.1093/ageing/25.4.285.
48. Sandberg L. Just feeling a naked body close to you: men, sexuality and intimacy in later life. Sexualities. 2013;16(3/4):261–82. https://doi.org/10.1177/1363460713481726.
49. Blumenstock SM, Quinn-Nilas C, Milhausen RR, McKay A. High emotional and sexual satisfaction among partnered midlife Canadians: associations with relationship characteristics, sexual activity and communication, and health. Arch Sex Behav. 2020;49(3):953–67. https://doi.org/10.1007/s10508-019-01498-9.
50. Roels R, Janssen E. Sexual and relationship satisfaction in young, heterosexual couples: the role of sexual frequency and sexual communication. J Sex Med. 2020;17(9):1643–52. https://doi.org/10.1016/j.jsxm.2020.06.013.
51. Gillespie BJ. Sexual synchronicity and communication among partnered older adults. J Sex Marital Ther. 2017;43(5):441–55. https://doi.org/10.1080/0092623X.2016.1182826.
52. Centers for Disease Control and Prevention (2018) Atlas Plus: HIV, hepatitis, STD, TB, social determines of health data. https://www.cdc.gov/nchhstp/atlas/index.htm.
53. Johnson BK. Sexually transmitted infections and older adults. J Gerontol Nurs. 2013;39(11):53–60. https://doi.org/10.3928/00989134-20130918-01.
54. Tillman JL, Mark HD. HIV and STI testing in older adults: an integrative review. J Clin Nurs. 2015;24(15–16):2074–95. https://doi.org/10.1111/jocn.12797.

55. Gott M, Hinchliff S, Galena E. General practitioner attitudes to discussing sexual health issues with older people. Soc Sci Med. 2004;58(11):2093–103. https://doi.org/10.1016/j.socscimed.2003.08.025.
56. Dogan S, Demir B, Eker E, Karim S. Knowledge and attitudes of doctors toward the sexuality of older people in Turkey. Int Psychogeriatr. 2008;20(5):1019–27. https://doi.org/10.1017/S1041610208007229.
57. Mahieu L, de Casterlé BD, Acke J, Vandermarliere H, Van Elssen K, Fieuws S, Gastmans C. Nurses' knowledge and attitudes toward aged sexuality in Flemish nursing homes. Nurs Ethics. 2016;23(6):605–23. https://doi.org/10.1177/0969733015580813.
58. Fürst J, Krall H. Sexualität – ein vernachlässigtes Thema in der psychodrama Ausbildung? [sexuality – a neglected topic in psychodrama training?]. Zeitschrift für Psychodrama und Soziometrie. 2012;11:25–39. https://doi.org/10.1007/s11620-012-0141-1.
59. Roberts M. Balint groups: a tool for personal and professional resilience. Can Fam Physician. 2012;58(3):245–7. https://www.ncbi.nlm.nih.gov/pubmed/22423015.
60. Barrett C. Auditing organisational capacity to promote the sexual health of older people. Electron J Appl Psychol. 2011;7(1):31–6. https://doi.org/10.7790/ejap.v7i1.233.
61. Watzlawick P, Beavin Bavelas J, Jackson D. Pragmatics of human communication - a study of interactional patterns, pathologies, and paradoxes. New York: W. W. Norton; 2011.
62. Lambert MJ, Barley DE. Research summary on the therapeutic relationship and psychotherapy outcome. Psychotherapy. 2001;38:357–61.
63. Rogers CR. The necessary and sufficient conditions of therapeutic personality change. J Consult Psychol. 1957;21(2):95–103.
64. Rogers CR, Farson RE. Active listening. Chicago: University of Chicago Industrial Relations Center; 1957.
65. Bachmair S, Faber J, Henning C, Kolb R, Willig W. Beraten will gelernt sein. Ein praktisches Lehrbuch für Anfänger und Fortgeschrittene. 3rd ed. Weinheim: Beltz; 1999.
66. Dahmer H, Dahmer J. Gesprächsführung. Eine praktische Anleitung. 4th ed. Stuttgart: Thieme; 1999.
67. Schulz von Thun F. Miteinander reden: Störungen und Klärungen. Allgemeine Psychologie der Kommunikation. Reinbek: Rowohlt; 1981.
68. Centers for Disease Control and Prevention (2005) A guide to taking a sexual history. https://stacks.cdc.gov/view/cdc/12303.

Future Directions for Research and Practice in Sexual Health for Older Adults

Igor Grabovac

13.1 Introduction

As the world's population is aging, older adults have become the fastest growing subpopulation. Between 1950 and 2017, the number of people aged 60 or older quadrupled. With further doubling projected over the next few decades, the world would see an estimated 2.1 billion people over the age of 60 by 2050 [1]. This demographic shift will create specific new challenges for policy makers given its expected impact on health and social systems. This was already made evident in the United Nation's report on an aging world in 2017, which promoted concepts such as active and healthy aging and mostly focused on prevention of noncommunicable diseases as well as mental and cognitive issues [2]. Despite ever-louder calls for a substantial "life course approach" [2], sexual health remains a so-called "topic of minimal interest" [3, 4]. Policy makers and health researchers tend to consider the topic taboo and often neglect the role that sexuality and intimacy play in quality of life in older adults and maintaining good health in older age [3]. Various chapters in this book detail both the role of sexuality, sexual activities, and intimacy as well as the reasons why they are neglected in research and healthcare of older adults. In this chapter, we will instead outline some of the foci that should be prioritized in the coming decades for better and broader inclusion in both research and practice of the sexual health of older adults. The following is an incomplete list of topics, which existing research and practice have brought to the forefront.

I. Grabovac (✉)
Department of Social and Preventive Medicine, Center for Public Health, Medical University of Vienna, Vienna, Austria
e-mail: igor.grabovac@meduniwien.ac.at

© Springer Nature Switzerland AG 2023
L. Smith, I. Grabovac (eds.), *Sexual Behaviour and Health in Older Adults*, Practical Issues in Geriatrics, https://doi.org/10.1007/978-3-031-21029-7_13

13.2 Prevention of Sexually Transmitted Infections in Older Adults

There is a considerable gap in the literature on epidemiological trends of sexually transmitted infections (STIs) in older adults. This is mostly connected to the fact that most national and international data gathering efforts do not extend after the age of 45 and also to the lack of routine assessments of sexual health in older adults by healthcare professionals [5]. However, the literature that does exist highlights higher vulnerability of older adults towards STIs. While the overall prevalence and incidence of STIs still seems to be low in older adults (compared to younger adults), some recent literature in the field suggests that overall numbers in this particular population group are indeed rising [5–7]. This may be due to lack of knowledge on measures for protection and prevention of STIs, or physiological issues such as vaginal dryness and erectile dysfunction (for more information see Chap. 7).

Setting *"Prevention of sexually transmitted infections"* as a priority for research in the field of sexual health in older adults is important not only from the point of establishing a good epidemiological overview of the situation, which will aid in creating the appropriate preventive programs targeting this population (and their evaluation), but it will also improve the visibility of these issues among healthcare practitioners which is urgently needed. Late presentation and recognition of STIs in older adults is well established as a problem for public health, leading to late therapeutic intervention detrimental for recovery as well as increasing risk of complications in individuals and spread of disease in the population. With regard to infections with the human immunodeficiency virus (HIV) and its treatment, more research is necessary on the effects of antiretroviral therapy (ART) in older patients, as some studies have recently shown slower response rates in patients over the age of 50 [8]. More so, even though ART has shifted HIV to a chronic lifelong condition, the effects of ART on the aging process is severely understudied and healthcare providers require more data to aid in prescribing the appropriate therapies to their older and aging patients [9].

13.3 Effects of Noncommunicable Diseases and Medication on Sexual Health of Older Adults

Chronic noncommunicable diseases show a rising prevalence in older adults, with multimorbidity—defined as having two or more chronic diseases concurrently—also rising with age. More than 60% of people over the age of 65 have two or more chronic diseases [10, 11]. Yet, good health is an important factor in maintaining sexual activity during the life course. Chronic physical and mental illness has an obvious effect on sexual activity in a large number of older adults. On the other hand, maintaining sexual activity throughout the life course also contributes to better health in later life [12, 13].

Policy makers should feel incentivized to focus more on the health issues of older adults given the demographic shift and the rising pressures it creates on health and social systems. However, the influence of chronic diseases and multimorbidity on sexual health and well-being in older adults is largely ignored in various policy work and international calls for active and healthy aging. While overall research in this field is lacking, existing studies have shown that chronic diseases and multimorbidity mediate sexual function by limiting physical function, reducing mobility, increasing pain, influencing mood and desire, as well as reducing self-esteem (for more information see Chap. 10). Chronic diseases and conditions such as arthritis, type II diabetes mellitus, cardiac disease, obesity, renal disorders, lung diseases, as well as prostate and ovarian cancer and more have all been associated with sexual dysfunction in older adults [14–16].

The rise in multimorbidity is usually followed by a rise in prescription medication. While these are often needed to maintain the health status and quality of life, older adults are under particularly high risk of receiving more than one prescription medication, often resulting in polypharmacy [17]. Prevalence of polypharmacy varies between countries and studies, but most studies report between 30% and 50% of older adults being prescribed 5 or more medications [18]. Some reports also note between 10% and 15% of older adults showing excessive polypharmacy (meaning the concomitant use of more than 10 medications) [19, 20]. While polypharmacy is a major public health concern as it may lead to dangerous therapeutic combinations and side effects, it may also pose a problem for the sexual health of older adults taking the medication (for more information see Chap. 9). While most healthcare practitioners are aware of this problem, the evidence on the effects of medication and their combinations on sexual function in older adults are largely anecdotal [21]. Sexual dysfunction is most commonly precipitated by the use of antihypertensive medication (beta-blockers and diuretics), antiandrogens, antipsychotics, and antidepressants, but more research in this field is crucial [21–23].

Given the virtual lack of evidence on the effects of chronic illness and medication use on sexual function in older adults, older adults need to be considered and included in clinical trials for new medication in a first instance [24]. However, questions on sexual activities, including experience of potential sexual dysfunction but also sexual satisfaction, are also paramount. Doing so will not only develop this field of research but will also be important for healthcare providers. Older adults do want and need information on sexual activity from their healthcare providers and show much of the same concerns as other patients in younger age groups (information on how to promote a positive atmosphere when talking to older adults on matters of sexual health in the clinic see Chap. 12).

13.4 Research Focusing on Sexual Satisfaction as Well as Positive Effects of Sexual Activity on Health of Older Adults

Overall, the majority of literature on the sexual health of older adults focuses on physiological and negative effects such as vaginal dryness, painful intercourse, anorgasmia, or erectile dysfunction. Only few studies focus either exclusively or additionally on sexual satisfaction. However, the topic of sexual satisfaction is of key importance for older adults as changes in physical functioning will also affect views and experiences of sex and sexuality. Sexual satisfaction is a highly individual concept that may be difficult to generalize. Overall, it may include positive feelings about one's body, arousal, pleasure, openness, and orgasm, but may also include relational factors such as intimacy, romance, creativity, and emotions among others [25]. Therefore, sexual health and having a "positive sex life" do not relate only to medical issues. Sexual health is personal; it has social, mental, and emotional aspects. More so, even though older adults still report relatively high activity in penetrative sex (vaginal and oral), considerations of sexual activity in older adults must also involve questions on kissing, fondling, (mutual) masturbation, and other activities. There are also differences in how men and women define having a "positive sex life," with men focusing more on the frequency of sexual intercourse and women more on enjoyment of intercourse. These factors have also been found to act as protective factors for premature mortality [26–31].

As noted above, good health is important for sexual activity, but sexual activity is also important for good health. Various studies have established that "frequent sexual intercourse" (equal to or more than twice a month) is associated with improved mental and physical health outcomes. Also, sexual activity—both in terms of intercourse and other activities such as kissing, fondling, and petting—has, for instance, been found to be associated with greater enjoyment of life in older adults in England [32].

It is important to create a safe environment with patients so sexuality can be openly discussed without stigmatization or stereotyping (for more see Chap. 12). This means likewise that future generations of healthcare practitioners need to be taught how to not only retrieve important medical information but also establish meaningful dialogue with their patients and provide them with enough and appropriate information so they can make informed decisions themselves. Such information will have to go beyond preventing or treating sexual dysfunction and include maintaining positive and satisfactory sexual lives far into older age.

13.5 Diversity Aspects in Research and Practice of Sexual Health of Older Adults

With the evidence base on various aspects of sexual health in older adults lacking overall, original research on diversity issues regarding the sexual health of older adults is no exception. The bulk of available research focuses almost exclusively on heterosexual cisgender older men. Moreover, most research in sexual health so far has focused on sexual dysfunction rather than salutogenetic aspects of sexual activity for overall health and well-being. Together, these foci have resulted in an overrepresentation of issues around erectile dysfunction in the literature.

More recently and in light of aspirations for more gender inclusivity in research, a number of articles and meta-analyses have focused on female sexual health—albeit, again, mostly on dysfunction rather than satisfaction. With regard to the latter, researchers have highlighted the effects of gender inequality in their reports on women's sexual satisfaction. For example, within the Global Study of Sexual Attitudes and Behaviours (2004) and an extensive dataset from 29 countries covering 27,500 men and women, researchers focused on four components of sexual health: satisfaction, physical pleasure, emotional pleasure, and importance of sex. The analyses exposed three different clusters or "sexual regimes": gender equal, mixed, and male-centered [33, 34]. These "regimes" highlighted differences in the way women rate their overall sexual satisfaction with their sexual function across regimes, with satisfaction being highest in "gender equal" regimes (median satisfaction 78%), moderate in "mixed" regimes (median satisfaction 56%), and lowest in "male-centered" regimes (median satisfaction 45%). Similar trends were also seen for other components analyzed. Even more interestingly, women had consistently lower scores across all three regimes compared to men, with differences being larger in more male-centered regimes [33]. These results were further validated by a meta-analysis in 2016 by McCool et al. [35], where a positive correlation between the prevalence of level of gender inequality and sexual dysfunction in women was also demonstrated. Upon further stratification, the authors also found that regions mostly situated in the Global North reported prevalence levels of female sexual dysfunction below 40%, with developing regions reporting rates higher than 62%. In light of the "regimes" identified in the 2004 Global Study, McCool et al. did not find significant differences with regard to sexual satisfaction. However, they did note lower rates of dyspareunia, difficulties with lubrication, and anorgasmia in "gender equal" regimes compared to "male-centered." In 2018, McCool-Myers [36] performed a systematic review update and a qualitative analysis of the results, and reported specific risk factors associated with sexual satisfaction in women in relation to the previously established "sexual regimes." Risk factors in countries with "gender equal sexual regimes" included cardiovascular disease, taking antidepressants, sleep problems, and polypharmacy, while in the "mixed" and "male-centered" regimes risk factors were mostly associated with early partnership and reproduction: young age at marriage, having an older partner, being in an arranged marriage, high number of births, but also nulliparity. They also reported unique predictors including genital mutilation, rural living, dieting, and restrictive upbringing. The study also found that most of the research from European and Western countries reveals a significant gap in the literature. Overall, older age, poor health, and relationship dissatisfaction were found to be significant predictors for female sexual dysfunction across all "sexual regimes." Even as more evidence is being gathered on the experiences of women and female sexuality, much more research is still needed that seriously takes into account socio-medical aspects of gender inequality that is context-specific.

Notably, none of the studies mentioned above include issues of sexual and gender diversity. While we could assume that all study participants are simply heterosexual cisgender men and women, the more likely explanation is that questions of sexual and gender diversity are not even posed during data collection. The reasons for this are multifaceted and may be due to prevalence of heterosexual participants in community-based studies or the reluctance of sexual and gender minorities to disclose their sexuality and gender identity to researchers. Yet, research must also be assumed to be inherently biased towards assuming heterosexuality and cisgenderism in participants [37, 38].

Lesbian, gay, bisexual, transgender, intersex, and queer people (LGBTIQ+) as a whole report worse physical and mental health outcomes compared to heterosexual and cisgender people [39]. Reasons for this vary, but one of the most prominent is minority stress due to stigma experienced for being nonheterosexual and/or transgendered. Minority stress is caused by (unwilling) nondisclosure of one's identity, as well as having experiences of discrimination, but also having internalized and anticipating discrimination [40, 41]. Living in hostile environments has been shown to be associated with worse health outcomes. A 2019 study by Grabovac et al. [42] analyzed cross-sectional data from the nationally representative English Longitudinal Study of Aging and reported that lesbian, gay, and bisexual older adults in England had lower quality of life scores and lower levels of sexual satisfaction compared to their heterosexual counterparts. Given the lack of data, however, no analyses were possible for transgender, nonbinary, or intersex individuals. Overall, some studies also report that gay men experience more ageism, and LGBTIQ+ people may be more at risk for loneliness and isolation due to their inability to live in legally recognized unions in most parts of the world. The ability to live in a legally recognized union has indeed been associated with less psychiatric morbidity and psychological distress [43–45]. In 2020, a cross-sectional study by Fleischmann et al. [46] reported that men and women aged 60–75 living in same-sex relationships showed high levels of relationship satisfaction and resilience, moderate levels of sexual satisfaction, and low levels of internalized homophobia. No other studies focusing on sexual activity or sexual satisfaction/dysfunction in older lesbian gay or bisexual individuals could be identified.

Older transgender individuals are even less present in the literature, with no studies at all available on aspects of sexual health in transgender older adults. However, a 2022 study using data from 325 participants of the ENIGI (European Network for the Investigation of Gender Incongruence) study did report, using the Amsterdam Sexual Pleasure Index, that younger age (as well as current happiness and genital body satisfaction) was associated with more sexual experiences of sexual pleasure, indicating that older adults experience less sexual pleasure [47]. Additionally, in a 2014 study by Friedriksen-Goldsen et al. [48] transgender older adults were found to be at a significantly higher risk for poor physical health, disability, depression, and stress compared to their cisgender counterparts. We may hypothesize that given the data indicating overall poorer health in transgender older adults, there is also a significant prevalence of sexual health issues and low sexual satisfaction. Finally, nonbinary and intersex people are virtually invisible in the literature concerning sexual health. With their experiences in the healthcare system being reportedly mostly unsatisfactory and problematic (high levels or stigmatization and discrimination), it is highly likely that the levels of dissatisfaction and poor health outcomes for intersex and nonbinary people are similarly high.

Beyond gender and sexual orientation, the relationship of physical disability and sexual health is significantly understudied. As levels of physical disability rise with age and multimorbidity, it is crucial to investigate the experiences of non-ablebodied older adults, and to create environments and techniques that would allow for satisfactory sexual activities. In a 2003 study by McCabe and Taleporos [49], 1196 people aged 18–69 were interviewed (60% having a physical disability). The authors report that people with more severe physical impairments experienced much lower levels of sexual self-esteem and satisfaction compared to those with milder forms of disability or no disability at all. A study on the use of aids for sexual activity in middle-aged adults with long-term physical disability did show that use of aids was generally associated with better sexual function, but this result varied by type of disability. Overall, the lowest levels of sexual satisfaction were found in men with spinal cord injury [50]. In 2003, Onder et al. [51] analyzed data from 980 women with moderate to severe disabilities aged 65 and older, using data from the 1992/1995 Women's Health and Aging Study. Their report showed that around 50% of women who lived with a spouse describe being satisfied with their sexual activity. Older age, being Caucasian, and having higher levels of physical functioning were shown to be associated with more sexual satisfaction. It is important to note that disability does not reduce desires for intimacy. However, due to harmful portrayals in the media and overall underrepresentation in research, stereotypes are created which often infantilize people with disability and propagate views of them as "asexual" [52]. Such stereotypes and biases need to be challenged by increasing, both in media and in research, the presence of people with disability. Only such, safe environments can be created where topics of sexual functioning and activity can be discussed with healthcare providers and the evidence is there to provide adequate care.

13.6 Making Sexual Health of Older People a Health Policy Priority

The demographic shift and rise of older adults as a subgroup within the world population have already incentivized international policy change that voices the needs of healthy aging. However, sexual health remains a "topic of minimal interest" for both researchers and practitioners. Where there is interest, it is usually focused on experiences of heterosexual and cisgender older men—less so, but also on women—and focuses mostly on medical issues and dysfunctions connected to penetrative sexual intercourse. This means that older adults rarely get the type of help they need from a healthcare system not designed for their sexual health needs and concerns.

The introduction of the Millennium Development Goals and Sustainable Development Goals, which both aim to ensure healthy lives and promote well-being of all ages, provided opportunity for the promotion of age-inclusive health and social systems that would provide a holistic view of older adults as patients [53, 54]. Ideally, this would include the sexual health needs of older adults, especially as they were recognized as significantly excluded from accessing appropriate sexual health services. However, little has changed so far [55].

To achieve change, effective strategies for large-scale epidemiological studies need to be created, with questions on both sexual health and practices routinely assessed. Beyond that, more qualitative work still needs to be done on the meaning of sex and sexuality, and so as to investigate both facilitators and barriers experienced by older adults. Furthermore, researchers, practitioners, and policy makers alike need to actively work to diminish the cultural stereotyping of older adults as being "asexual" or "celibate," and to promote healthy and positive views of sexuality in older age. This societal shift dovetails recent research showing that older adults today are much more open on topics of sex and sexual activity than the generations before them. Such changes might be expedited if researchers, practitioners, and policy makers took a clear stance.

13.7 Final Remarks

There is much work to be done in research on the sexual health of older adults. More attention needs to be afforded to the life experiences of older adults, and how sexuality and sexual activity fit into them. This means both the experiences of sex and sexuality of older adults with multimorbidity and chronic illness, but also an understanding of older adults as a very diverse group. Older adults are people of various gender identities and expressions, sexual orientations, ethnicities, socioeconomic status, religious beliefs, and more. All of it affects sexual activity and sexual health. More research should result in more advocacy work and policy change to reflect the needs of older adults, provide appropriate access, and assure that they get the help they need from their healthcare providers. The sexual health of older adults must therefore be included as a key topic in the training of future healthcare professionals and in courses for the continuous education of practitioners already working.

The above list is neither exhaustive nor complete and presents only the opinion of its author and his limited research experience. The list should be viewed as signposts to highlight the areas where more work is desperately needed, while keeping in mind that the sexual health of older adults is, as a whole, still underresearched or not properly understood.

References

1. United Nations Department of Economic and Social Affairs Population Division. World population ageing - highlights (ST/ESA/SER.A/397). New York: United Nations; 2017.
2. World Health Organization. Multisectoral action for a life course approach to healthy aging: draft global strategy and plan of action on ageing and health 2016 [cited 2022 29.07.2022]. https://apps.who.int/gb/ebwha/pdf_files/WHA69/A69_17-en.pdf?ua=1.
3. Aboderin I. Sexual and reproductive health and rights of older men and women: addressing a policy blind spot. Reprod Health Matters. 2014;22(44):185–90. https://doi.org/10.1016/S0968-8080(14)44814-6.
4. World Health Organization Regional Office for Europe. The life course approach: from theory to practice. Case stories from two small countries in Europe. Geneva: World Health Organization Regional Office for Europe; 2018.
5. Poynten IM, Grulich AE, Templeton DJ. Sexually transmitted infections in older populations. Curr Opin Infect Dis. 2013;26(1):80–5. https://doi.org/10.1097/QCO.0b013e32835c2173.

6. Bodley-Tickell AT, Olowokure B, Bhaduri S, White DJ, Ward D, Ross JDC, et al. Trends in sexually transmitted infections (other than HIV) in older people: analysis of data from an enhanced surveillance system. Sex Transm Infect. 2008;84(4):312–7. https://doi.org/10.1136/sti.2007.027847.
7. Wang C, Zhao P, Xiong M, Tucker JD, Ong JJ, Hall BJ, et al. New syphilis cases in older adults, 2004–2019: an analysis of surveillance data from South China. Front Med (Lausanne). 2021;8:781759. https://doi.org/10.3389/fmed.2021.781759.
8. Balestre E, Eholié SP, Lokossue A, Sow PS, Charurat M, Minga A, et al. Effect of age on immunological response in the first year of antiretroviral therapy in HIV-1-infected adults in West Africa. AIDS. 2012;26(8):951–7. https://doi.org/10.1097/QAD.0b013e3283528ad4.
9. Esteban-Cantos A, Rodríguez-Centeno J, Barruz P, Alejos B, Saiz-Medrano G, Nevado J, et al. Epigenetic age acceleration changes 2 years after antiretroviral therapy initiation in adults with HIV: a substudy of the NEAT001/ANRS143 randomised trial. Lancet HIV. 2021;8(4):e197–205. https://doi.org/10.1016/S2352-3018(21)00006-0.
10. Ofori-Asenso R, Lee Chin K, Curtis AJ, Zomer E, Zoungas S, Liew D. Recent patterns of multimorbidity among older adults in high-income countries. Popul Health Manag. 2019;22(2):127–37. https://doi.org/10.1089/pop.2018.0069.
11. Salive ME. Multimorbidity in older adults. Epidemiol Rev. 2013;35:75–83. https://doi.org/10.1093/epirev/mxs009.
12. Addis IB, Van Den Eeden SK, Wassel-Fyr CL, Vittinghoff E, Brown JS, Thom DH, et al. Sexual activity and function in middle-aged and older women. Obstet Gynecol. 2006;107(4):755–64. https://doi.org/10.1097/01.AOG.0000202398.27428.e2.
13. Lindau ST, Gavrilova N. Sex, health, and years of sexually active life gained due to good health: evidence from two US population based cross sectional surveys of ageing. BMJ. 2010;340:c810. https://doi.org/10.1136/bmj.c810.
14. Camacho ME, Reyes-Ortiz CA. Sexual dysfunction in the elderly: age or disease? Int J Impot Res. 2005;17(Suppl 1):S52–6. https://doi.org/10.1038/sj.ijir.3901429.
15. Ni Lochlainn M, Kenny RA. Sexual activity and aging. J Am Med Dir Assoc. 2013;14(8):565–72. https://doi.org/10.1016/j.jamda.2013.01.022.
16. Palacios S, Castano R, Grazziotin A. Epidemiology of female sexual dysfunction. Maturitas. 2009;63(2):119–23. Epub 2009/06/02. https://doi.org/10.1016/j.maturitas.2009.04.002.
17. Masnoon N, Shakib S, Kalisch-Ellett L, Caughey GE. What is polypharmacy? A systematic review of definitions. BMC Geriatr. 2017;17(1):230. https://doi.org/10.1186/s12877-017-0621-2.
18. Pazan F, Wehling M. Polypharmacy in older adults: a narrative review of definitions, epidemiology and consequences. Eur Geriatr Med. 2021;12(3):443–52. https://doi.org/10.1007/s41999-021-00479-3.
19. Morin L, Johnell K, Laroche ML, Fastbom J, Wastesson JW. The epidemiology of polypharmacy in older adults: register-based prospective cohort study. Clin Epidemiol. 2018;10:289–98. https://doi.org/10.2147/CLEP.S153458.
20. Salvi F, Rossi L, Lattanzio F, Cherubini A. Is polypharmacy an independent risk factor for adverse outcomes after an emergency department visit? Intern Emerg Med. 2017;12(2):213–20. https://doi.org/10.1007/s11739-016-1451-5.
21. Thomas DR. Medications and sexual function. Clin Geriatr Med. 2003;19(3):553–62. https://doi.org/10.1016/s0749-0690(02)00101-5.
22. Segraves RT, Balon R. Antidepressant-induced sexual dysfunction in men. Pharmacol Biochem Behav. 2014;121:132–7. https://doi.org/10.1016/j.pbb.2013.11.003.
23. Taylor MJ, Rudkin L, Bullemor-Day P, Lubin J, Chukwujekwu C, Hawton K. Strategies for managing sexual dysfunction induced by antidepressant medication. Cochrane Database Syst Rev. 2013;(5):CD003382. https://doi.org/10.1002/14651858.CD003382.pub3.
24. Herrera AP, Snipes SA, King DW, Torres-Vigil I, Goldberg DS, Weinberg AD. Disparate inclusion of older adults in clinical trials: priorities and opportunities for policy and practice change. Am J Public Health. 2010;100 Suppl 1:S105–12. https://doi.org/10.2105/AJPH.2009.162982.

25. Pascoal PM, Narciso Ide S, Pereira NM. What is sexual satisfaction? Thematic analysis of lay people's definitions. J Sex Res. 2014;51(1):22–30. https://doi.org/10.1080/00224499.2013.815149.
26. Brody S, Preut R. Vaginal intercourse frequency and heart rate variability. J Sex Marital Ther. 2003;29(5):371–80. https://doi.org/10.1080/00926230390224747.
27. Costa RM, Brody S. Sexual satisfaction, relationship satisfaction, and health are associated with greater frequency of penile-vaginal intercourse. Arch Sex Behav. 2012;41(1):9–10. https://doi.org/10.1007/s10508-011-9847-9.
28. Ebrahim S, May M, Ben Shlomo Y, McCarron P, Frankel S, Yarnell J, et al. Sexual intercourse and risk of ischaemic stroke and coronary heart disease: the Caerphilly study. J Epidemiol Community Health. 2002;56(2):99–102. https://doi.org/10.1136/jech.56.2.99.
29. Flynn TJ, Gow AJ. Examining associations between sexual behaviours and quality of life in older adults. Age Ageing. 2015;44(5):823–8. https://doi.org/10.1093/ageing/afv083.
30. Heiman JR, Long JS, Smith SN, Fisher WA, Sand MS, Rosen RC. Sexual satisfaction and relationship happiness in midlife and older couples in five countries. Arch Sex Behav. 2011;40(4):741–53. https://doi.org/10.1007/s10508-010-9703-3.
31. Palmore EB. Predictors of the longevity difference: a 25-year follow-up. Gerontologist. 1982;22(6):513–8. https://doi.org/10.1093/geront/22.6.513.
32. Smith L, Yang L, Veronese N, Soysal P, Stubbs B, Jackson SE. Sexual activity is associated with greater enjoyment of life in older adults. Sex Med. 2019;7(1):11–8. https://doi.org/10.1016/j.esxm.2018.11.001.
33. Laumann EO, Paik A, Glasser DB, Kang JH, Wang T, Levinson B, et al. A cross-national study of subjective sexual well-being among older women and men: findings from the global study of sexual attitudes and behaviors. Arch Sex Behav. 2006;35(2):145–61. https://doi.org/10.1007/s10508-005-9005-3.
34. Nicolosi A, Laumann EO, Glasser DB, Moreira ED Jr, Paik A, Gingell C, et al. Sexual behavior and sexual dysfunctions after age 40: the global study of sexual attitudes and behaviors. Urology. 2004;64(5):991–7. https://doi.org/10.1016/j.urology.2004.06.055.
35. McCool ME, Zuelke A, Theurich MA, Knuettel H, Ricci C, Apfelbacher C. Prevalence of female sexual dysfunction among premenopausal women: a systematic review and meta-analysis of observational studies. Sex Med Rev. 2016;4(3):197–212. https://doi.org/10.1016/j.sxmr.2016.03.002.
36. McCool-Myers M, Theurich M, Zuelke A, Knuettel H, Apfelbacher C. Predictors of female sexual dysfunction: a systematic review and qualitative analysis through gender inequality paradigms. BMC Womens Health. 2018;18(1):108. https://doi.org/10.1186/s12905-018-0602-4.
37. DeLamater J. Sexual expression in later life: a review and synthesis. J Sex Res. 2012;49(2–3):125–41. https://doi.org/10.1080/00224499.2011.603168.
38. Institute of Medicine. The health of lesbian, gay, bisexual, and transgender people: building a foundation for better understanding. Washington, DC: The National Academies Press; 2011. p. 366.
39. Emlet CA. Social, economic, and health disparities among LGBT older adults. Generations. 2016;40(2):16–22.
40. Meyer IH. Prejudice, social stress, and mental health in lesbian, gay, and bisexual populations: conceptual issues and research evidence. Psychol Bull. 2003;129(5):674–97. https://doi.org/10.1037/0033-2909.129.5.674.
41. Wight RG, LeBlanc AJ, de Vries B, Detels R. Stress and mental health among midlife and older gay-identified men. Am J Public Health. 2012;102(3):503–10. https://doi.org/10.2105/AJPH.2011.300384.
42. Grabovac I, Smith L, McDermott DT, Stefanac S, Yang L, Veronese N, et al. Well-being among older gay and bisexual men and women in England: a cross-sectional population study. J Am Med Dir Assoc. 2019;20(9):1080–5.e1. https://doi.org/10.1016/j.jamda.2019.01.119.
43. Hatzenbuehler ML, McLaughlin KA, Keyes KM, Hasin DS. The impact of institutional discrimination on psychiatric disorders in lesbian, gay, and bisexual populations: a prospective study. Am J Public Health. 2010;100(3):452–9. https://doi.org/10.2105/AJPH.2009.168815.

44. Kail BL, Acosta KL, Wright ER. State-level marriage equality and the health of same-sex couples. Am J Public Health. 2015;105(6):1101–5. https://doi.org/10.2105/AJPH.2015.302589.
45. Riggle ED, Rostosky SS, Horne SG. Psychological distress, well-being, and legal recognition in same-sex couple relationships. J Fam Psychol. 2010;24(1):82–6. https://doi.org/10.1037/a0017942.
46. Fleishman JM, Crane B, Koch PB. Correlates and predictors of sexual satisfaction for older adults in same-sex relationships. J Homosex. 2020;67(14):1974–98. https://doi.org/10.1080/00918369.2019.1618647.
47. Gieles NC, van de Grift TC, Elaut E, Heylens G, Becker-Hebly I, Nieder TO, et al. Pleasure please! Sexual pleasure and influencing factors in transgender persons: an ENIGI follow-up study. Int J Transgender Health. 2022:1–13. https://doi.org/10.1080/26895269.2022.2028693.
48. Fredriksen-Goldsen KI, Cook-Daniels L, Kim HJ, Erosheva EA, Emlet CA, Hoy-Ellis CP, et al. Physical and mental health of transgender older adults: an at-risk and underserved population. Gerontologist. 2014;54(3):488–500. https://doi.org/10.1093/geront/gnt021.
49. McCabe MP, Taleporos G. Sexual esteem, sexual satisfaction, and sexual behavior among people with physical disability. Arch Sex Behav. 2003;32(4):359–69. https://doi.org/10.1023/a:1024047100251.
50. Smith AE, Molton IR, McMullen K, Jensen MP. Brief report: sexual function, satisfaction, and use of aids for sexual activity in middle-aged adults with Long-term physical disability. Top Spinal Cord Inj Rehabil. 2015;21(3):227–32. https://doi.org/10.1310/sci2103-227.
51. Onder G, Penninx BW, Guralnik JM, Jones H, Fried LP, Pahor M, et al. Sexual satisfaction and risk of disability in older women. J Clin Psychiatry. 2003;64(10):1177–82. https://doi.org/10.4088/jcp.v64n1006.
52. Milligan MS, Neufeldt AH. The myth of asexuality: a survey of social and empirical evidence. Sex Disabil. 2001;19(2):91–109. https://doi.org/10.1023/A:1010621705591.
53. Elias C, Sherris J. Reproductive and sexual health of older women in developing countries. BMJ. 2003;327(7406):64–5. https://doi.org/10.1136/bmj.327.7406.64.
54. United Nations Development Programme. Sustainable development goals 2022 [cited 2022 28.07.2022]. https://www.undp.org/sustainable-development-goals.
55. Banke-Thomas A, Olorunsaiye CZ, Yaya S. "Leaving no one behind" also includes taking the elderly along concerning their sexual and reproductive health and rights: a new focus for reproductive health. Reprod Health. 2020;17(1):101. https://doi.org/10.1186/s12978-020-00944-5.

Concluding Summary

14

Igor Grabovac and Lee Smith

People are living longer. While differences in life expectancy still exist between countries, older adults make up a group of growing numbers, both relative and absolute, all around the world. Recent projections suggest that 2.1 billion people will be over the age of 60 in 2050, which is already twice the number of 2022 [1]. Aging, as a process, is associated with a variety of biological changes and their buildup, which lead to increased risk for various diseases and death. Beyond the biological, aging is also associated with a variety of social and psychological changes such as retirement, the death of friends and partners, taking on a less active role in society, and so on. An aging population also delivers new challenges to health and social systems given a rise in multimorbidity and increased healthcare utilization. However, aging can also be an opportunity, as the availability of more time to spare can provide older adults with a chance to pursue new activities often neglected while part of the active workforce or due to familial obligations. To live full and engaged lives far into older age, older adults need the support from their political, medical, and social environments. Barriers need to be removed and opportunities created to facilitate healthy activities that promote good health and well-being in older age [1].

One of the most important and most neglected aspects inextricably linked to good health and well-being is sexuality. Sexuality is complex and encompasses a number of different dimensions, such as partnership, behaviors, attitudes, identity, orientation, and activity [2]. Culturally, sex and sexuality are often seen solely as means for reproduction, associated with youth and fertility. This often leads to misconceptions of sex and sexuality of older adults and a general lack of positive

---

I. Grabovac (✉)
Department of Social and Preventive Medicine, Center for Public Health, Medical University of Vienna, Vienna, Austria
e-mail: igor.grabovac@meduniwien.ac.at

L. Smith
Centre for Health, Perform and Wellbeing, Anglia Ruskin University, Cambridge, UK
e-mail: lee.smith@anglia.ac.uk

representations of sex among older adults. On the other hand, such stereotypes are coupled with a significant rise in the production and marketing of pharmaceuticals aimed at managing sexual dysfunction for both older men and women. Even if not commonly discussed in either communities, clinics, or among researchers, this fact does indeed suggest that older adults are sexually active and considered to be sexually active—at least by the market. The field of research on sexual activities and sexual health in older adults is still small, but a growing international push is palpable for more original studies to elucidate the question: *what is needed for good sex in older age,* and *how do people have good sex in older age*?

In defining sexual health, the World Health Organization (WHO) notes that *"it is a state of physical, emotional, mental, and social well-being in relation to sexuality and not only an absence of disease, dysfunction or infirmity."* Furthermore, the WHO emphasizes the need of an open and positive approach focused on safe and pleasurable sexual experiences, free of discrimination and coercion, which can only be achieved if sexual rights of people are respected, protected, and fulfilled [3]. This can only be achieved through policy changes based on scientific evidence and good clinical practice, to which this book is making a small but significant contribution.

Across its chapters, the book has established that sexual activity persists during the life course. While a marked decline is noticeable in the frequency of sexual activities with age, sexual activity is still maintained. In an influential epidemiological study of over 27,000 men and women aged 40 to 80, more than 80% of men and 65% of women reported being sexually active in the past year [4]. Even studies with very old adults, those aged between 85 and 95, showed that almost one third still engaged in sexual activities [5, 6]. Most common activities include vaginal sex, which remains the most frequent form of sexual activity reported among 80% of older men and 75% of older women [2, 7]. It is important to note that sexual activity, and especially sexual activity in older age, encompasses more than penetrative sex and does also involve touching, petting, (mutual) masturbation, sharing phantasies, and emotionality overall. Additionally, data on sexual activities and sexuality in older adults provides almost exclusively insights on heterosexual and cisgender people, limiting the generalizability of these results and their consideration of diversity aspects.

Overall, studies have demonstrated the link between sexual activity and physical health [8–10]. As aging is associated with a range of physiological changes, these also include changes in the reproductive system, mostly associated with hormonal changes more expressive—from a physiological standpoint—in women rather than men. These changes may lead to sexual dysfunction both physiological—such as decreased vaginal lubrication, dyspareunia, or erectile dysfunction—and also psychological, including reduced libido, changes in mood and in self-esteem. Age also increases the prevalence of chronic illness which mediates sexual function through limited physical function, pain, or by lowering self-esteem. Health is important to maintain sexual activities in older age, but sexual activity is also associated with better health in later life. For example, a study from the English Longitudinal Study of Aging reported that those older adults, who reported a decline in frequency of sexual activities, had higher chances of also experiencing limited long-standing illness and reported overall deterioration of self-reported health [11]. In a cross-sectional study in the United States of 22,654 adults over the age of 55, results indicated that sexual inactivity was associated with cancer, bladder or bowel issues, major surgery, poor vision, mental health conditions, but also cardiovascular disease and more [12].

An active sexual life has also been connected to better mental health and quality of life. A 2019 study done in the United Kingdom found that men and women, who reported having had any sexual activity in the past year, also had significantly higher scores for enjoyment of life compared to those who did not report any sexual activity [13]. Similar studies have also noted the relationship between sexual activity and quality of life as well as overall well-being [14, 15]. Just as with physical health, the relationship between mental health and sexual health in older adults appears to be bidirectional. Studies have confirmed that older adults with better mental health also report more satisfaction with sexual activities [16]. Mental health disorders, such as depression, are associated with reported sexual problems among older adults [17]. The same can be said for anxiety, especially the anxiety about the ability to perform sexually, as well as body image issues and low self-esteem [18].

Sexuality in older age is also influenced by social conditions and characteristics of the community in which one lives. For example, some studies have shown that, as people age, their social networks change. This may influence their sexual lives, as the most important factor for engaging in sexual activities is being able to find a partner. Therefore, it is not surprising that one study reported that 70% of older women and 38% of older men reported that the main reason for their sexual inactivity was the lack of a partner [19]. Beyond diminishing social networks, social forces also shape sexual experiences of older adults through stigma and the image of the "sexless" older person. A study by Waterman in 2012 [20] showed that college students showed more surprise and disgust when reading a text on sexual activity between people who were 70–75 compared to protagonists 30–35 years old. They also found sexual activity between people in their 70s to be less acceptable and appropriate. Also, as previously noted, almost all studies on sexual activities and sexuality in older adults stem from data on cisgender and heterosexual participants. However, some more recent studies have already highlighted that older lesbian, gay, and bisexual people report lower levels of sexual satisfaction compared to their heterosexual counterparts [21]. As far as we can assume, the situation of transgender and nonbinary individuals may even be worse. There is virtually no literature on their sexual health or satisfaction, but selected studies have indeed suggested that older age is associated with less sexual satisfaction in transgender people. Even more worryingly, few healthcare professionals exhibit the cultural competence and are trained to navigate diversity issues in order to offer adequate counseling and treatment to lesbian, gay, bisexual, transgender, intersex, and queer (LGBTIQ+) older adults [22].

Given the myriad of positive effects of sex and sexuality on overall health and well-being, it is necessary for healthcare practitioners to adequately address potential negative issues and corresponding factors. More specifically, healthcare providers need to be acutely aware of the barriers that older people face and which are unique to this population. Basic knowledge and evidence about the sexual activity and sexuality of older adults is required so as to enable healthcare professionals to openly and easily talk about sex and sexuality with their older patients [23]. Sexuality is multifaceted and complex. Broaching topics of sexual function and sexual lives in older patients demands the capacities of an interdisciplinary team composed of physicians and psychologists, as well as physiotherapists and occupational therapists to provide a holistic and well-rounded approach to older patients and clients.

14.1 Concluding Remarks

This book is a small contribution to a slowly growing field on sexual health in older adults. It is our hope that it will provide readers a good overview of the current evidence base and future generations of interested researchers a place from which to launch new ideas and future projects. As such, it will be interesting to students of the health sciences and medicine, as well as researchers focused on aging or sexuality. Moreover, the authors of individual chapters were asked to give, where available, a practical overview. The book should therefore also lend a hand in approaching topics of sexuality with older patients for those working in the clinical field—geriatricians, urologists, gynecologists, general practitioners, and mental health experts alike. Lastly, given that many chapters focus on community and societal aspects of sexuality in older adults, the book encompasses dimensions of sexuality that would be equally interesting to professionals working in disease prevention, health promotion, and gerontology.

We thank all the authors for their selfless contributions. We would especially like to express our gratitude to Professor Daragh T. McDermott, who provided invaluable input and feedback as the associate editor for this book.

References

1. World Health Organization. Ageing and health 2021 [cited 2022 27.07.2022]. https://www.who.int/news-room/fact-sheets/detail/ageing-and-health.
2. Lindau ST, Schumm LP, Laumann EO, Levinson W, O'Muircheartaigh CA, Waite LJ. A study of sexuality and health among older adults in the United States. N Engl J Med. 2007;357(8):762–74. https://doi.org/10.1056/NEJMoa067423.
3. World Health Organization. Sexual health 2022 [cited 2022 25.07.2022]. https://www.who.int/health-topics/sexual-health#tab=tab_2.
4. Nicolosi A, Laumann EO, Glasser DB, Moreira ED Jr, Paik A, Gingell C, et al. Sexual behavior and sexual dysfunctions after age 40: the global study of sexual attitudes and behaviors. Urology. 2004;64(5):991–7. https://doi.org/10.1016/j.urology.2004.06.055.
5. Hyde Z, Flicker L, Hankey GJ, Almeida OP, McCaul KA, Chubb SA, et al. Prevalence of sexual activity and associated factors in men aged 75 to 95 years: a cohort study. Ann Intern Med. 2010;153(11):693–702. https://doi.org/10.7326/0003-4819-153-11-201012070-00002.

6. Lindau ST, Gavrilova N. Sex, health, and years of sexually active life gained due to good health: evidence from two US population based cross sectional surveys of ageing. BMJ. 2010;340:c810. https://doi.org/10.1136/bmj.c810.
7. Waite LJ, Laumann EO, Das A, Schumm LP. Sexuality: measures of partnerships, practices, attitudes, and problems in the National Social Life, Health, and Aging Study. J Gerontol B Psychol Sci Soc Sci. 2009;64 Suppl 1:i56–66. https://doi.org/10.1093/geronb/gbp038.
8. Brody S, Preut R. Vaginal intercourse frequency and heart rate variability. J Sex Marital Ther. 2003;29(5):371–80. https://doi.org/10.1080/00926230390224747.
9. Friedman S. Cardiac disease, anxiety, and sexual functioning. Am J Cardiol. 2000;86(2, Supplement 1):46–50. https://doi.org/10.1016/S0002-9149(00)00893-6.
10. Miner M, Esposito K, Guay A, Montorsi P, Goldstein I. Cardiometabolic risk and female sexual health: the Princeton III summary. J Sex Med. 2012;9(3):641–51; quiz 52. https://doi.org/10.1111/j.1743-6109.2012.02649.x.
11. Jackson SE, Yang L, Koyanagi A, Stubbs B, Veronese N, Smith L. Declines in sexual activity and function predict incident health problems in older adults: prospective findings from the English longitudinal study of ageing. Arch Sex Behav. 2020;49(3):929–40. https://doi.org/10.1007/s10508-019-1443-4.
12. Bach LE, Mortimer JA, VandeWeerd C, Corvin J. The association of physical and mental health with sexual activity in older adults in a retirement community. J Sex Med. 2013;10(11):2671–8. https://doi.org/10.1111/jsm.12308.
13. Smith L, Yang L, Veronese N, Soysal P, Stubbs B, Jackson SE. Sexual activity is associated with greater enjoyment of life in older adults. Sex Med. 2019;7(1):11–8. https://doi.org/10.1016/j.esxm.2018.11.001.
14. Flynn TJ, Gow AJ. Examining associations between sexual behaviours and quality of life in older adults. Age Ageing. 2015;44(5):823–8. https://doi.org/10.1093/ageing/afv083.
15. Jackson SE, Firth J, Veronese N, Stubbs B, Koyanagi A, Yang L, et al. Decline in sexuality and wellbeing in older adults: a population-based study. J Affect Disord. 2019;245:912–7. https://doi.org/10.1016/j.jad.2018.11.091.
16. Matthias RE, Lubben JE, Atchison KA, Schweitzer SO. Sexual activity and satisfaction among very old adults: results from a community-dwelling Medicare population survey. Gerontologist. 1997;37(1):6–14. https://doi.org/10.1093/geront/37.1.6.
17. Schreiner-Engel P, Schiavi RC. Lifetime psychopathology in individuals with low sexual desire. J Nerv Ment Dis. 1986;174(11):646–51. https://doi.org/10.1097/00005053-198611000-00002.
18. Ni Lochlainn M, Kenny RA. Sexual activity and aging. J Am Med Dir Assoc. 2013;14(8):565–72. https://doi.org/10.1016/j.jamda.2013.01.022.
19. Smith LJ, Mulhall JP, Deveci S, Monaghan N, Reid MC. Sex after seventy: a pilot study of sexual function in older persons. J Sex Med. 2007;4(5):1247–53. https://doi.org/10.1111/j.1743-6109.2007.00568.x.
20. Waterman EA. Reactions of college students to the sexuality of older people. J Student Res. 2012;1(2):46–50. https://doi.org/10.47611/jsr.v1i2.54.
21. Grabovac I, Smith L, McDermott DT, Stefanac S, Yang L, Veronese N, et al. Well-being among older gay and bisexual men and women in England: a cross-sectional population study. J Am Med Dir Assoc. 2019;20(9):1080–5.e1. https://doi.org/10.1016/j.jamda.2019.01.119.
22. Knochel KA, Croghan CF, Moone RP, Quam JK. Training, geography, and provision of aging services to lesbian, gay, bisexual, and transgender older adults. J Gerontol Soc Work. 2012;55(5):426–43. https://doi.org/10.1080/01634372.2012.665158.
23. Fürst J, Krall H. Sexualität – ein vernachlässigtes Thema in der Psychodrama Ausbildung? Zeitschrift für Psychodrama und Soziometrie. 2012;11(1):25–39. https://doi.org/10.1007/s11620-012-0141-1.

Glossary

15

Lisa Lehner and Charlotte Rösel

The following glossary provides an overview and short definitions of key terminology used in this book. It is meant as an accessible on-hand reference for the reader. For more information and details, please consult appropriate textbooks and up-to-date scientific literature.

Term	Definition
Ageism	Ageism refers to the *stereotypes* [*see stereotype*], prejudice, and *discrimination* [*see discrimination*] towards others or oneself on the basis of age
Anabolism	Anabolism is the building-up mechanism of the metabolism in living cells and organisms. Anabolic processes are enzyme-catalyzed reactions by which relatively complex molecules are formed from smaller and relatively simple molecules. *Opp.* catabolism
Anorgasmia	Anorgasmia describes the absence of attaining orgasm after sufficient sexual stimulation. Anorgasmia is associated with significant personal distress and *sexual dissatisfaction* [*see satisfying sex, sexual fulfillment*]
Arousal (sexual)	Arousal (sexual) refers to the physiological and psychological processes in the body when exposed to sexual stimuli (e.g., touch, mental stimuli, physical stimuli, internal fluctuation of hormones)

L. Lehner (✉) · C. Rösel
Department of Social and Preventive Medicine, Centre for Public Health, Medical University of Vienna, Vienna, Austria
e-mail: lisa.lehner@meduniwien.ac.at

Term	Definition
Asexuality	An asexual person is someone who does not experience sexual attraction. A person who is asexual can experience attraction that can be romantic, aesthetic, or sensual; they might experience *arousal* [see arousal (sexual)], *desire* [see desire (sexual)], or seek romantic relationships. The split attraction model helps to express both sexual and romantic attraction of people who identify as asexual and experience romantic attraction to different *genders* [see gender]. If people identify as asexual and experience romantic attraction to the same gender, they might identify as asexual *homoromantic* or asexual and *lesbian or gay* [see homosexual, gay, lesbian]. Asexuality describes a spectrum of disinclination towards sexual behavior or sexual partnering
Bisexuality	Bisexuality describes a person's capacity to form romantic, sexual, or emotional attraction towards people presenting both as *male* [see male] and *female* [see female], or to more than one *gender* [see gender]. People who identify as bisexual need not experience equal attraction across genders
Cisgender	Cisgender (or cis*) describes a person whose *gender identity* [see sexual and gender identity] corresponds to their *gender* [see gender] assigned at birth. *Opp. transgender* [see transgender]
Cisnormativity	Cisnormativity describes the implicit and systemic assumption that all, or almost all, people are *cisgender* [see cisgender]
Comorbidity	Comorbidity describes the presence of one or more additional conditions often co-occurring (concomitant or concurrent) with a primary condition
Cultural setting	A cultural setting describes a place, space, or institution in which a social group can be said to share a set of (implicit and explicit) values, ideas, concepts, and rules of behavior. Culture cannot be said to be present or absent, but such values, ideas, rules, and concepts are dynamic, evolving, and socially constructed by the members of a social group
Desire (sexual)	Sexual desire describes a conscious impulse towards someone or something that promises (sexual) enjoyment or satisfaction in its attainment
Discrimination	Discrimination is the unfair or prejudicial treatment of individual people or groups based on characteristics such as *gender identity* [see sexual and gender identity], race, age, dis/ability, sexual orientation, mental health, and others
Disempowerment	Disempowerment describes processes by which individual people or social groups are actively or structurally denied, deprived of, or inhibited in their agency, authority, influence, or ability to make choices and succeed
Dysfunction	Dysfunction describes impaired or abnormal functioning (e.g., of biochemical bodily responses during sexual intercourse)
Dyslipidemia	Dyslipidemia refers to an elevation of plasma cholesterol, triglycerides, or both, or a low high-density lipoprotein cholesterol level that contributes to the development of atherosclerosis; causes may be primary (genetic) or secondary
Dyspareunia	Dyspareunia refers to painful intercourse for physiological and/or psychological reasons that occurs just before, during, or after sex
External stressors	External stressors refer to stress-inducing processes that occur in a person's surroundings or environment. *Opp.* internal stressors
Female	Relating to or characteristic of behaviors, appearances, interests, etc. traditionally associated with the biologically female sex; having a *gender identity* [see sexual and gender identity] that is the opposite of *male* [see male]

15 Glossary

Term	Definition
Fondling	To touch gently and in a loving way, or to touch in a sexual way
Frailty; pre-frailty	Older adults with chronic conditions, decreased physical function, and cognitive impairment are more likely to become frail, which negatively affects their *quality of life* [see *quality of life*] and life expectancy. Frailty is a multifactorial syndrome resulting in increased *vulnerability* [see *vulnerable group*] to adverse outcomes that is associated with malnutrition, inadequate physical activity, hormonal imbalance, multimorbidity, and detrimental socioeconomic conditions. Frailty is associated with a prodromal stage called pre-frailty, a potentially reversible condition before onset of established frailty
Gatekeeper	Gatekeeper describes a person who has the power to actively or implicitly decide or inhibit access to opportunities, resources, or spaces for another person or group
Gay	Gay describes the sexual orientation, attraction, and *self-identification* [see *self-identification*] of people who are emotionally, romantically, and/or physically attracted to people of the same *gender* [see *gender*]. Gay often refers specifically to the attraction of people who identify as *male* [see *male*] to people who also identify as male. *Lesbian* [see *lesbian*] is often a preferred term for attraction between people who identify as *female* [see *female*]
Gender	A social combination of identity, expression, and social elements related to masculinity and femininity. Gender includes different aspects, such as *sexual and gender identity* [see *sexual and gender identity*] (*self-identification* [see *self-identification*]), gender expression (self-expression), social gender (social expectations), *gender roles* [see *gender role*] (socialized actions), and gender attribution (social perception)
Gender minority	Gender minority generally refers to groups with *gender identities* [see *sexual and gender identity*] and expressions which differ from the numerical majority. Being in the gender minority often relates to the gender binary. The gender binary refers to the cultural insistence and idea that there are only two *genders* [see *gender*], either *male* [see *male*] or *female* [see *female*], and the assumption that gender is biologically determined. People who identify as neither male or female, both, or something else are generally considered to be in the minority. The status of being in the minority is often related to *marginalization* [see *marginalization*], *discrimination* [see *discrimination*], and *stigma* [see *stigma*] (*minority stress* [see *minority stress*])
Gender reassignment surgery	Gender reassignment surgical procedures help people *transition* [see *transition*] to their *self-identified gender* [see *gender, self-identification*] and may include facial surgery, top surgery, or bottom surgery. Today, reassignment surgeries are also often referred to as gender affirmation or gender confirmation surgeries
Gender roles	The behaviors, attitudes, values, beliefs, etc. which a social group or culture consider appropriate for a *male* [see *male*] or *female* [see *female*] person
Global life satisfaction	Global life satisfaction is the cognitive component of subjective well-being and is defined as an individual's appraisal of their overall *quality of life* [see *quality of life*]
Hegemony	Hegemony is the political, economic, social, and/or cultural predominance of one state or group over others

Term	Definition
Heteronormativity	Heteronormativity describes the implicit and systemic assumption that all, or almost all, people fall into distinct genders (*male* [*see male*] or *female* [*see female*]), and naturalizes *heterosexual* [*see heterosexual*] coupling of a *man* [*see man*] with a *woman* [*see woman*] as the norm
Heterosexism	Heterosexism describes prejudice against people and groups who display *non-heterosexual* [*see heterosexuality*] behaviors or identities, combined with the majority power to impose such a prejudice
Heterosexuality	Heterosexuality describes a person's romantic, emotional, and sexual attraction towards a different *gender* [*see gender*] than their own
Homophobia	Homophobia refers to an implicit or express aversion to people who identify as *homosexual* [*see homosexuality*], *gay* [*see gay*], or *lesbian* [*see lesbian*] which often manifests as prejudice, bias, *discrimination* [*see discrimination*], stigma [*see stigma*], or violence [*see sexual violence*]. Similarly, biphobia might refer specifically to an aversion against people who identify as bisexual [*see bisexuality*]. Collectively, these attitudes are referred to as *anti-LGBTIQ+ bias* [*see LGBTIQ+*]
Homosexuality	Homosexuality describes a person's same-gender romantic, emotional, and sexual attraction; primary use of the term is clinical, and use of more specific terms is preferred, such as *gay* [*see gay*], *lesbian* [*see lesbian*], or *queer* [*see queer*]
Internalization	Internalization refers to a process of socialization into a given society or culture, through which external norms, rules, attitudes, values, and biases become (implicitly) accepted by an individual and thus internal. Terms such as internalized *homophobia* [*see homophobia*] or internalized *stigma* [*see stigma*] describe a person's acceptance of dominant biases against their own (minority) *sexual or gender identity* [*see sexual and gender identity*], which might be exhibited as self-hatred or self-denial
Intimacy	Intimacy refers to physical and/or emotional closeness, or feelings of closeness (e.g., during sexual intercourse)
Lesbian	Lesbian describes the sexual orientation, attraction, and *self-identification* [*see self-identification*] of people who are emotionally, romantically, and/or physically attracted to people of the same *gender* [*see gender*], whereby the term specifically refers to the attraction of people who identify as *female* [*see female*] to people who also identify as female
LGBTIQ+	An acronym that collectively refers to people who identify as *lesbian* [*see lesbian*], *gay* [*see gay*], *bisexual* [*see bisexuality*], *trans** [*see transgender*], *inter**, or *queer* [*see queer*], or *questioning* [*see questioning*]. Different versions of the acronym exist that include or exclude certain sexual and gender orientations and identities [*see sexual and gender identity*]. The plus sign aims to create greater inclusivity and represents any non-*heterosexual* [*see heterosexuality*] and non-cis* [*see cisgender*] identity not expressly included
Libido	Libido describes a person's overall sexual drive or *desire* [*see desire (sexual)*] for *sexual activity* [*see sexual activity*]
Lust	Lust usually refers to intense or unbridled sexual *desire* [*see desire (sexual)*]
Male	Relating to or characteristic of behaviors, appearances, interests, etc. traditionally associated with the biologically male sex; having a *gender identity* [*see sexual and gender identity*] that is the opposite of female [*see female*]
Man	Man generally describes a human person who currently identifies as *male* [*see male*], lives as a man, or identifies predominantly as masculine

15 Glossary

Term	Definition
Marginalization	Marginalization describes an implicit or express social process by which a person or group are considered or made to be insignificant or peripheral to the norm or numerical majority
Minority stress	The minority stress model was first theorized in the context of research on the mental health of people who identify as *LGBTIQ+* [*see LGBTIQ+*]. It intends to express the greater social stresses faced by people who identify as a sexual or *gender minority* [*see gender minority*], such as homophobia [*see homophobia*] and *discrimination* [*see discrimination*]. Such stresses leave numerical minorities at higher risk for substance use and negative mental health outcomes, including depressive symptoms and suicide ideation
Monogamy	Monogamy is the practice or state of having a sexual relationship with only one partner
MSM	*Men* [*see man*] who have sex with men
Nondisclosure	Nondisclosure is used to refer to the (intentional) act of not revealing one's own *queer identity* [*see queer, gender identity*] in a particular context. Nondisclosure is often a person's choice and does not mean they are deceiving anyone
Partnered sex	Partnered sex involves one or more partners for the purpose of sexual pleasure [*see pleasure (sexual)*]. *Sexual activity* [*see sexual activity*] and sexual behaviors can, but must not, involve partners (auto-eroticism)
Penile inversion vaginoplasty	Penile inversion vaginoplasty is a technique of *gender reassignment genital surgery* [*see gender reassignment surgery*] that uses primarily genital skin to construct the vulva and neovagina for patients assigned *male* [*see male*] at birth
Petting	Engaging in sexually stimulating caressing and touching
Plateau (sexual)	The plateau phase of sexual bodily response describes the highest point of *sexual pleasure* [*see pleasure (sexual)*] and continues to grow, lasting several seconds to minutes. A person may feel physical and emotional excitement and have physical sensations of sensitivity and warmth
Pleasure (sexual)	*Noun*: a feeling of happy satisfaction and enjoyment, also in the context of sexual intercourse or auto-eroticism; *verb:* give sexual enjoyment or *satisfaction* to someone [*see satisfying sex*] or to oneself
Polypharmacy	Polypharmacy is often defined as the routine use of five or more medications; includes over-the-counter, prescription, and/or traditional and complementary medicines used by a patient
Quality of life	Quality of life (or QOL) refers to the standard of health, comfort, and happiness experienced by a person or group; different measures and measurements are used to assert quality of life
Queer	An umbrella term representative of the vast matrix of identities outside of the cisgender [*see cisgender*] and *heterosexual* [*see heterosexuality*] majority; reclaimed after a history of pejorative use, starting in the 1980s; may also be used as a term for self-identification [*see self-identification*]
Questioning	Questioning refers to a process of exploration by a person who might be unsure, still exploring, or concerned about their sexual or gender self-identification [*see sexual and gender identity, self-identification*], expression, or sexual orientation
Reproductive health	Reproductive health is a state of complete physical, mental, and social well-being and not merely the absence of disease or infirmity, in all matters relating to the reproductive system and to its functions and processes. Reproductive health implies that people are able to have a *satisfying* [*see satisfying sex*] and *safe* [*see safe sex techniques*] sex life, and that they have the capability to reproduce and the freedom to decide if, when, and how often to do so

Term	Definition
Safe sex techniques	Safe sex techniques refer to acts or behaviors that reduce the risk of infection with a sexually transmitted disease [see *STIs*] (e.g., the use of condoms)
Sarcopenia	Sarcopenia is a type of muscle loss (muscle atrophy) that occurs with aging and/or immobility. It is characterized by the degenerative loss of skeletal muscle mass, quality, and strength
Satisfying sex	Satisfying sex or a satisfying sex life will vary from person to person. Sexual satisfaction may refer to or include quality and frequency of sexual activity [see *sexual activity*], arousal [see *arousal (sexual)*], or orgasm, mutual pleasure [see *pleasure (sexual)*], acting out of desires [see *desire (sexual)*], or partnership satisfaction
Self-identification	Self-identification refers to the assigning of a particular characteristic or categorization to oneself, often used to describe self-identification with a particular *gender* [see *gender*] or sexual orientation. Self-identification is the key measure by which sexual and gender identity [see *sexual and gender identity*], attraction, and sexual orientation can be asserted
Self-revelation	Self-revelation refers to the process by which a person's *gender identity* [see *sexual and gender identity*] or sexual orientation become known to themselves over time. The term assumes the self to be fluid and socially constructed; it supplants the negatively connotated term self-deception
Sexual activity; sexual conduct	Sexual activity describes the manner in which people experience and express their sexuality
Sexual and gender identity	Sexual and gender identity describes an individual's internal sense of being *male* [see *male*], *female* [see *female*], both, neither (agender), or something else (genderqueer, genderfluid, gender non-conforming, etc.)
Sexual assault	Sexual assault is an act of intentionally touching another person, or coercing or forcing another person to engage in a sexual act without that person's express and repeated consent. Sexual assault is a form of *sexual violence* [see *sexual violence*]. Legal definitions of sexual assault may differ across countries and settings
Sexual culture	Sexual culture may refer to a set of rules, norms, values, and behaviors shared by a social group or subgroup related to sexuality, *sexual activity*, and *sexual conduct* [see *sexual activity*]
Sexual expression	Sexual expression is used to refer to the expression of sexual desire [see *desire (sexual)*] and sexual acts with a diverse and expansive understanding of human sexuality that goes beyond cisnormative [see *cisnormativity*] and heteronormative [see *heteronormativity*] assumptions of penile-vaginal intercourse among male-female dyads [see *male, female*]. Continued sexual expression in older age is increasingly researched and connected to greater sexual and overall health
Sexual fulfillment	Sexual fulfillment refers to the state of satisfaction with one's sexual life [see *satisfying sex*] and sexuality
Sexual function	Sexual function is how the body reacts in different stages of the sexual response cycle, or as a result of sexual dysfunction [see *dysfunction*]
Sexual health	Sexual health requires a positive and respectful approach to sexuality and sexual relationships, as well as the possibility of having pleasurable [see *pleasure (sexual)*] and safe [see *safe sex techniques*] sexual experiences, free of coercion, discrimination [see *discrimination*] and violence [see *sexual violence*]

15 Glossary

Term	Definition
Sexual rights	Under international human rights law, all persons have the right to control and decide freely on matters related to their sexuality; to be free from violence [see *sexual violence*], coercion, or intimidation in their sexual lives; to have access to sexual and reproductive healthcare information [see *sexual health, reproductive health*], education, and services; and to be protected from discrimination [see *discrimination*] based on the exercise of their sexuality
Sexual violence	Sexual violence is defined as a sexual act that is committed or attempted by another person without freely given consent or against someone who is unable to consent or refuse. Sexual violence is a comprehensive term that may refer to different forms of violence, such as rape, sexual assault [see *sexual assault*], sexual abuse, intimate partner sexual violence, incest, sexual harassment, elder abuse, and more. Sexual violence can also occur when a perpetrator forces or coerces someone to engage in sexual acts with a third party. Sexual violence can occur to anybody at any age
SGM	Sexual and gender minority (SGM) communities include, but are not limited to, individuals who identify as *lesbian* [see *lesbian*], *gay* [see *gay*], *bisexual* [see *bisexuality*], *asexual* [see *asexuality*], *transgender* [see *transgender*], Two-Spirit, *queer* [see *queer*], inter*, or, more generally, any *sexual and gender identity* [see *sexual and gender identity*] that does not fit into cis* [see *cisnormativity*], hetero [see *heteronormativity*], or monogamous [see *monogamy*] social norms
Social attachment	Within attachment theory, attachment means an affectional bond or tie between an individual and an attachment figure (usually a caregiver); different attachment styles formed during childhood are generally assumed to be expressed as distinct patterns in adult relationships
Social background	Social background generally refers to the totality of socially transmitted behaviors, attitudes, values, beliefs, institutions, and biases that a person has grown up in and belongs to; background may refer more specifically to a person's social class, education, cultural and ethnic belonging, nationality, or similar
Social passivity	Social passivity refers to persons' passivity in the initiating, forming, and/or maintaining of social relationships
Social well-being	Social well-being describes a person's—especially an older person's—good health related to the presence and quality of their social relationships, their social networks, their social participation/loneliness, sexuality, social support, caregiver burden, and general social environment
Societal acceptance	Societal acceptance refers to the implicit and express mechanisms of inclusion, especially of *minority groups* [see *gender minority*] into the social majority; societal acceptance can be considered on a spectrum ranging from tolerating to active inclusion
SRA-Q ELSA	Sexual relationships and activities questionnaire (SRA-Q) of the English longitudinal study of ageing (ELSA)
Stereotype	Stereotypes refer to a widely held but fixed and oversimplified image or idea of a particular type of person, group, thing, or concept
Stigma	Stigma refers to a social mark of disgrace associated with a particular circumstance, quality, or person; stigmatization describes the process by which or state of a person who is stigmatized for a particular characteristic, identity, or quality by society or a group
STIs	Sexually transmitted infections, such as HIV (human immunodeficiency virus), syphilis, or herpes simplex virus; STIs are spread predominantly by sexual contact, including vaginal, anal, and oral sex

Term	Definition
Successful aging	Successful aging has become an important concept to describe the quality of the aging process. It is a multidimensional concept with the main focus on how to expand functional years during the later life span. The concept has developed from a biomedical approach to a wider understanding of social and psychological adaptation processes in later life
Taboo	Prohibited or restricted by social custom
Transgender	Transgender (or trans*) describes a person whose *gender identity* [see *sexual and gender identity*] does not necessarily correspond to their *gender* [see *gender*] assigned at birth and may be used as an umbrella term to denote the wide variety of identities within the gender variant spectrum. The asterisk is representative of the widest notation of possible trans* identities. Other terms commonly used are *female-to-male* (or FTM), *male-to-female* (or MTF) [see *male, female*], assigned male at birth (or AMAB), assigned female at birth (or AFAB), genderqueer, nonbinary, genderfluid, or gender expansive. A person who identifies as transgender may choose to alter their bodies hormonally and/or surgically to match their gender identity through *gender affirmation surgery* [see *gender reassignment surgery*], or by socially *transitioning* [see *transition*] in various ways. *Opp. cisgender* [see *cisgender*]
Transition	The process by which some people strive to more closely align their *self-identified gender* [see *self-identification, gender*] with its outward appearance. Some people socially transition, whereby they might begin expressing, dressing, using names and pronouns, and/or being socially recognized as another gender. Others undergo physical transitions in which they modify their bodies through medical interventions (e.g., through gender affirmation surgery [see *gender reassignment surgery*])
Transphobia	Transphobia refers to an implicit or express aversion to people who identify as *transgender* [see *transgender*] which often manifests as prejudice, bias, *discrimination* [see *discrimination*], stigma [see *stigma*], or violence, *sexual* and otherwise [see *sexual violence*]
Vaginal atrophy	Vaginal atrophy (atrophic vaginitis) describes the thinning, drying, and inflammation of the vaginal walls that may occur when the body has less estrogen. Vaginal atrophy occurs most often after menopause. For many people with vaginas, vaginal atrophy not only makes intercourse painful [see *dyspareunia*] but also leads to distressing urinary symptoms
Vulnerable group	A group of persons may be more or less vulnerable to shock, ill-health, social and biological risks, social and natural hazards, and death due to a variety of social, natural, political, and economic conditions. A group's or person's state of vulnerability can be assessed across different dimensions: e.g., the initial level of well-being, the degree of exposure to risk, and the capacity to manage risk effectively. Vulnerability can be considered as both a condition and a process. Dynamic interactions between material and social deprivation, poverty, powerlessness, or health impacts may change, alleviate, or reinforce each other over time
Woman	Woman generally describes a human person who currently identifies as *female* [see *female*], lives as a woman, or identifies predominantly as feminine

Printed in the United States
by Baker & Taylor Publisher Services